Assessment of antenatal and obstetric care services
in a rural district of Nepal

Medizin in Entwicklungsländern

Schriftenreihe zur Medizin und zu Gesundheitsproblemen
in Ländern der Dritten Welt

Herausgegeben von
Prof. Dr. med. Hans Jochen Diesfeld, Heidelberg

Band 45

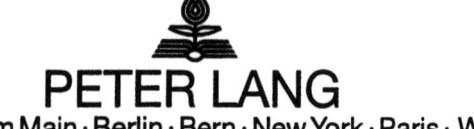

PETER LANG
Frankfurt am Main · Berlin · Bern · New York · Paris · Wien

Maureen Dar Iang

Assessment of antenatal and obstetric care services in a rural district of Nepal

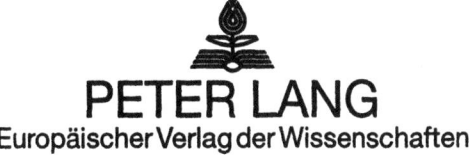

PETER LANG
Europäischer Verlag der Wissenschaften

Die Deutsche Bibliothek - CIP-Einheitsaufnahme

Dar Iang, Maureen:

Assessment of antenatal and obstetric care services in a rural district of Nepal / Maureen Dar Iang. - Frankfurt am Main ; Berlin ; Bern ; New York ; Paris ; Wien : Lang, 1999
(Medizin in Entwicklungsländern ; Bd. 45)
Zugl.: Heidelberg, Univ., Diss., 1997
ISBN 3-631-34718-9

This document is printed with the financial support
of German Academic Exchange Service
(Deutscher Akademischer Austauschdienst, DAAD), Bonn.

D 16
ISSN 0721-3247
ISBN 3-631-34718-9
US-ISBN 0-8204-4328-X

© Peter Lang GmbH
Europäischer Verlag der Wissenschaften
Frankfurt am Main 1999
All rights reserved.

All parts of this publication are protected by copyright. Any utilisation outside the strict limits of the copyright law, without the permission of the publisher, is forbidden and liable to prosecution. This applies in particular to reproductions, translations, microfilming, and storage and processing in electronic retrieval systems.

Table of Contents

List of tables	xii
List of figures	xiii
List of abbreviations	xiv
Forward by Prof. H. J. Diesfeld	xv
Acknowledgements	xvii
Executive summary	xix

1	Introduction	1- 3

1.1 The purpose of the study	2
1.1.1 The study questions	2
1.1.2 The study objectives	3

2	Literature review	5-28

2.1 Introduction	5
2.2 Nepal: the country background	5
2.2.1 Geography and demography	5
2.2.2 Politics, economy and society	6
2.2.3 The health care system	6
2.2.4 Nepal's safe motherhood policy and programme	7
The national antenatal risk catalogue	8
2.3 The global safe motherhood programme	9
2.3.1 The concept and goal of the global safe motherhood initiative	9
2.3.2 The history of safe motherhood programmes	10
2.3.3 The criticisms on safe motherhood programmes	11
2.3.3.1 Antenatal care	11
2.3.3.2 Obstetric care	12
2.3.3.3 Post-natal care and family planning	14
2.4 Assessing antenatal and obstetric care services	14
2.4.1 Definition of quality and methodological issues in quality assessment	15

2.4.2 Assessment of quality of antenatal and obstetric care service 17
    2.4.2.1 Availability 18
    2.4.2.2 Accessibility 18
        Geographical accessibility 19
        Financial accessibility 20
        Socio-cultural accessibility 20
    2.4.2.3 Coverage (utilisation) 21
    2.4.2.4 Performance of health services (service quality) 22
    2.4.2.5 Users satisfaction 24
2.4.3 Assessment of community perspectives on care during pregnancy and childbirth 25
    2.4.3.1 Beliefs and practices of community regarding pregnancy and childbirth 25
    2.4.3.2 Risk perception and perception of illness aetiology by community regarding pregnancy and childbirth 26
    2.4.3.3 Value and status of women in the society ... 27
    2.4.3.4 Perspectives of community on modern health services 28

2.5 Summary of literature on assessing safe motherhood programmes 28

| 3 | Material and Methods | 29-42 |

3.1 Introduction 29

3.2 Short description of the study area 29

3.3 Study design 29
    3.3.1 Study methods and data sources 29
    3.3.2 Study targets and selection of health facilities 30

3.4 Data collection 31
    3.4.1 Selection and training of interviewers 32
    3.4.2 Pilot testing 33
    3.4.3 Data collection instruments 33
    3.4.4 Quantitative data collection 34

Table of contents

	3.4.4.1 Document reviews	34
	3.4.4.2 Inventories of building, equipment, drugs and consumable	36
	3.4.4.3 Observation of health worker's performance	36
	3.4.4.4 Interviews with health workers	37
	3.4.4.5 Interviews with health service users	38
	Antenatal exit interviews	38
	Maternity interviews	38
3.4.5	Qualitative data collection	39
	3.4.5.1 Focus group discussions	39
	3.4.5.2 Key-informant interviews	40
3.5	Feedback to the community	41
3.6	Data recording and analysis	41
3.7	Limitations	42

4	Results	43-84

4.1	The state of maternal health care infrastructure in Banke district, Nepal	43
	4.1.1 Availability of antenatal and obstetric care services in the district	43
	4.1.1.1 Service outlets	43
	4.1.1.2 Health manpower	44
	Professional health workers	44
	Trained traditional birth attendants	44
	4.1.2 Availability of antenatal and obstetric care services in the selected facilities	45
	4.1.2.1 Health service outlets	45
	4.1.2.2 Health manpower	46
	4.1.2.3 Availability of essential equipment, drugs and consumable in the selected 14 FLHS	46
	4.1.2.4 Availability of equipment, drugs and consumable in the referral hospital	46
	4.1.3 Accessibility of antenatal and obstetric care services	48
	4.1.3.1 Geographical accessibility	48
	Geographical accessibility of selected 14 FLHS	48

		Geographical accessibility of referral level obstetric care	49
	4.1.3.2	Financial accessibility	50
		Financial accessibility of antenatal care services	50
		Financial accessibility of hospital delivery care services	51
	4.1.3.3	Socio-cultural accessibility	51
4.2	The state of maternal health care delivery in Banke district		51
	4.2.1	Coverage of maternal health care	52
	4.2.1.1	Antenatal care	52
		Antenatal coverage by FLHS and by distance	52
		Coverage by age and parity	52
		Coverage by religion	52
		Intensity of use	52
		Timeliness of care	53
	4.2.1.2	Delivery care	54
		Obstetric coverage by place of origin	55
		Obstetric coverage by age and parity	55
	4.2.1.3	Post-natal care	56
	4.2.2	Health service performances	56
	4.2.2.1	Knowledge of health workers excluding TBA	57
	4.2.2.2	Performance of health workers on preventive and promotive activities of ANC	58
		Consultation and counselling time	58
		Health education and counselling	58
		Effectiveness of health education and counselling	59
		Anaemia prophylactics	59
		Tetanus prophylactics	60
	4.2.2.3	Health worker's performance on screening activities	61
		Health worker's perception of high risk pregnancies	61
		History taking and examination	62
		Identification and correct interpretation of high risk pregnancies	62
		Sensitivity of the screening process	64

Table of contents

	4.2.2.4 Intervention according to risk factors and health problems identified: referral to referral level hospital	64
	Reasons for referral advice	64
	Population based referral advice rate of high risk pregnancies	64
	Referral compliance	65
	4.2.2.5 Management at referral level obstetric care ...	66
	Care at admission, delivery and discharge ...	67
	Timeliness of care	68
	Output related to obstetric care at referral level	68
	Coverage of high risk pregnancies at referral level	68
4.2.3	Outcome of maternal health care in referral level	70
	4.2.3.1 Stillbirth rate	70
	4.2.3.2 Maternal mortality ratio	71
4.2.4	Co-ordination and supervision among health workers	71
4.2.5	In-service training of health workers	71
4.3.6	Community involvement in health care delivery	71

4.3 Determinants of maternal health care services utilisation ... 72
    4.3.1 Quality of service according to service users 72
        Waiting time 72
        Reasons for choosing this centre 73
        Reasons for coming to ANC 73
        Reasons for intended hospital or home delivery 73
        Claimed benefits from antenatal care 74
        Patient satisfaction 75
        Suggestions 75
    4.3.2 Beliefs and practices of community regarding pregnancy and childbirth 75
        Nutrition 75
        Clean delivery 76
        Hard working and rest 76
        Sexual behaviour 77
        Medical intervention 77
    4.3.3 Risk perception by community regarding pregnancy and childbirth 77

4.3.4   Choice of healers according to beliefs on illness
         aetiology 77
         Vomiting and loss of appetite in pregnancy ... 78
         STD-related symptoms 78
         Retained placenta 79
         Prolonged labour 79
         High fever 80
4.3.5   Determinants of use of modern health service in 80
         pregnancy and childbirth ....
         4.3.5.1   The influence of cultural tradition on use of
                   services 80
                   Pregnancy and delivery seen as a natural
                   process 80
                   Childbirth as a family event 81
                   Shyness and fear 81
                   Social status of health workers 81
         4.3.5.2   The influence of health service factors 82
                   Relatively new services 82
                   Performance of health workers 82
                   Hospital regulations which do not consider
                   cultural value 82
                   Expensive hospital fees vs. Free service by
                   local healers 82
                   Organisational and geographical accessibility 83
         4.3.5.3   The influence of to socio-economic conditions
                   on use of service 83
                   Lack of education 83
                   Distribution of property and power 84

5	Discussion, conclusion and recommendations	85-106

5.1   Infrastructure and organisation of maternal health care   85
      services ....
5.2   Utilisation of antenatal and obstetric care services in Banke
      district 86
5.3   Why is the utilisation of maternity care services
      comparatively low in Banke district? 88
      5.3.1   Health service factors influencing utilisation 89

5.3.2	Does socio-cultural tradition play an important role in utilisation of modern maternity care services in Banke district?	92
5.4	Do preventive and promotive activities in antenatal care benefit antenatal attendees?	95
	Health education and counselling	95
	Prevention and treatment of anaemia	96
	Prevention of tetanus	96
5.5	Does risk approach in antenatal care work in this district?	97
	The process of screening, identification of risk pregnancy, and referral advice	97
	Management at referral level	100
5.6	Conclusion	101
	Socio-cultural factors play an important role in health services utilisation in this community	102
	Conventional deficiency of health service is impeding utilisation of health care services	102
	Low effectiveness of services for users	103
5.7	Recommendations	104

Bibliography **107-119**

List of annexes and maps **121-156**

List of Tables

Table	Title	Page
Table 1	Sampling frame with selected facilities and their catchment population	29
Table 2	Availability of health manpower, Banke district	45
Table 3	Availability of essential drugs and consumable at selected 14 FLHS	47
Table 4	Individual achievement of selected FLHS on drugs and supplies and on equipment for antenatal and delivery care	48
Table 5	Availability of essential equipment, drugs and consumable at labour room and theatre, government hospital	48
Table 6	Geographical accessibility of selected 14 FLHS	49
Table 7	Distance vs. means of transport used by antenatal attendees	49
Table 8	Accessibility of referral level hospital, Banke district	50
Table 9	Coverage of antenatal care by individual FLHS	53
Table 10	Antenatal coverage by age of women in selected 14 FLHS	53
Table 11	Antenatal coverage by number of gestation in selected 14 FLHS	54
Table 12	Weeks of gestation at 1st antenatal visit from AN card review	54
Table 13	Coverage of delivery by health care providers, Banke district	55
Table 14	Coverage of hospital delivery and population based CS rate by distance, Banke district	55
Table 15	Coverage of hospital delivery by age	56
Table 16	Coverage of hospital delivery by number of gestations	56
Table 17	Contents of health education given to antenatal attendees	59
Table 18	Health worker's perception of high risk pregnancies	61
Table 19	Essential contents of history taking, physical examination and laboratory tests done during antenatal care	63
Table 20	Reasons given for referral advice according to antenatal attendees and recorded in antenatal cards	65

Table 21	Availability of essential obstetric care at government hospital	67
Table 22	Profile of CS by indication, government & private hospitals	69
Table 23	Frequency of risk factors among hospital deliveries and pregnant women in the population, government hospital	69
Table 24	Stillbirth rate by mode of delivery, government hospital	70
Table 25	Still birth rate vs. place of origin & mode of delivery among hospital deliveries, government hospital	70
Table 26	Stillbirth rate by birth weight among vaginal delivery, government hospital	71
Table 27	Reasons given for choosing this centre for antenatal care	73
Table 28	Reasons given for intending hospital delivery by antenatal attendees	74
Table 29	Reasons given for intending home delivery by antenatal attendees	74
Table 30	Suggestions given to improve services by antenatal attendees	75

List of figures

Figure	Title	Page
Figure 1	Knowledge of FLHS staff on antenatal and obstetric care	57
Figure 2	Proportion of antenatal attendees counselled	58
Figure 3	Population based coverage of anaemia prophylactics in pregnancy	60
Figure 4	Effectiveness of screening in pregnancy, Banke district	66

List of Abbreviations

ANC	Antenatal Care
ANM	Auxiliary Nurse Midwife
APH	Ante-Partum Haemorrhage
BP	Blood Pressure
CS	Caesarean Section
DDC	District Development Committee
DMO	District Medical Officer
DPHO	District Public Health Officer
EOC	Essential Obstetric Care
FCHV	Female Community Health Volunteer
FLHS	First Line Health Service
GNP	Gross National Product
HDP	Hypertensive Diseases of Pregnancy
HIV	Human Immuno-deficiency Virus
HMG	His Majesty's Government
HP	Health Post
HW	Health Worker
LB	Live Birth
MCH	Maternal and Child Health
MCHW	Maternal Child Health Worker
MMR	Maternal Mortality Ratio
MoH	Ministry of Health
NFHS	Nepal Family Health Survey
OR	Odd Ratio
PHC	Primary Health Centre
PNMR	Perinatal Mortality Rate
PMMN	Prevention of Maternal Mortality Network
PPH	Post-Partum Haemorrhage
SB	Stillbirth
SHP	Sub-Health Post
STD	Sexually Transmitted Diseases
TBA	Traditional Birth Attendant
TT	Tetanus Toxoid
UNFPA	United Nations Association for Population Fund
UNICEF	United Nations Children's Fund
VDC	Village Development Committee
WHO	World Health Organisation

Foreword

After half a century of development efforts and in spite of all knowledge and skills available even in economically disadvantaged countries, like Nepal, motherhood is anything but safe.

Pregnancy and childbirth related morbidity and mortality is still appallingly high in spite of many antenatal and obstetric care concepts developed over the decade. Yet it is still one of the most important "unfinished agendas" of the ambitious goal "health for all". M for mother in MCH (Mother and Child Health Care) has been neglected for a long time.

WHO only recently has started to propagate "safe motherhood initiatives" and yet in the World Health Report 1998 WHO hardly mentions the dimension of this problem, let alone gives a clue how to overcome it.

Reasons for this unacceptable state of affairs are usually known: Many individual, communication and service related problems are mentioned. Complications in pregnancy and childbirth are only partially predictable or preventable. Swift and competent medical intervention is often the only chance for a favourable pregnancy outcome.

A prerequisite for safe motherhood is the too long neglected operational research in health care management for optimal utilisation of available skills and knowledge under unfavourable conditions.

Safe motherhood implies not only readily available intervention strategies and good quality of care. It requires also early detection of risk, followed by appropriate action, this in turn requires a good understanding and awareness of the risks and the chances for safe motherhood management, by the families of the mother as well as by the health services.

This study in Nepal has successfully developed an algorithm for the assessment of antenatal care and obstetric services in rural Nepal, taking service related variables, accessibility, acceptability and peoples perception of safe motherhood and risks into account.

The Nepal example can serve as a model approach to a comprehensive methodology for the assessment of antenatal and obstetric care as a contribution towards safer motherhood.

H. J. Diesfeld

Acknowledgements

For the successful completion of this document, many persons helped me from the preparation to the field study and the writing processes. As we forget many things in life, it is not possible to remember all who have contributed to this piece of work. I am most grateful to all those who have contributed, helped and shown interest in my work.

I am most grateful to Prof. H. J. Diesfeld, my doctor father, for encouraging me to write this document and your continuous fatherly support and guidance.

I am most grateful to Dr. Albrecht Jahn, my close supervisor. You give me endless assistance, guidance and support. I always appreciate your patience, understanding, and friendship.

I am most grateful to many persons in Nepal who contributed to make my field study to be feasible and fruitful. I would like to start my special thank with personnel from the STD/HIV project in Kathmandu, for your assistance and support. In Nepalganj Dr. M. Kidwai (DMO), Mr. Ratnalal Shrestha (DPHO), Dr. Usha Shah, Dr. G. R. Shakya and all personnel from the DMO's and the DPHO's offices, you supported us and accommodated us in your daily routines. I have no words to express my gratitude to Annette de Graaf, Erik Nijland, and family Ratan Man Shrestha through you we enjoyed our stay in Nepalganj.

The travelling, organising and conducting interviews were not an easy job for Sunila Shrestha, Razmi Shrestha, Kovita Kurung, and Champa Shrestha. I would like to thank you for your efforts and patience.

My special gratitude goes to all interviewees for sharing with me your knowledge and experiences.

Many thanks to Dr. Pitt Reitmaier, Dr. Sigrid Wolter, Ms. Anne Erpelding and all the staff of the ATHÖG for your support; Hajo Zeeb and Karina Kielmann for improving my English.

My special thanks to German Academic Exchange Service (DAAD), Bonn, for your financial support of my study as well as publication of this document.

I am most grateful to Marga, my friend. I always appreciate your endless assistance, friendship, and love. I can only appreciate and admire you, Jutta and family Flemming, through you our stay in Germany becomes a happy event to remember.

Finally my appreciation to you, my little daughter Stephanie. You give me enduring love and support.

Executive Summary

This study describes the situation of maternal health care services in Banke, a rural district of Nepal. It aims to assess and contribute to the improvement of quality of antenatal and obstetric care services. The starting point was concern about the high maternal and perinatal mortality (maternal mortality ratio 539/100,000 live births, perinatal mortality rate 57/1000 births), coinciding with a particularly low utilisation of maternal health care services in Nepal.

The quality of maternity services was assessed with a set of quantitative indicators. This was complemented by a community-based study on local risk concepts, perceived quality of care and other factors determining the use of modern health services in pregnancy and childbirth. Both qualitative and quantitative methodologies were applied. The data were collected in two hospitals and 14 first line health facilities and their catchment population. The data sources include: (1) document review covering 1378 first antenatal consultations and 1323 hospital deliveries; (2) inventories of staff, essential equipment, drugs and supplies in the selected health facilities; (3) interviews with health workers (n=19), health service users (antenatal attendees n=136, hospital deliveries n=146), and key-informants (n=21); and (4) 6 focus group discussions (56 participants).

Health infrastructure

Banke district has 42 first line health facilities serving a population of 338,000 (1 facility per 8000 population). However, antenatal care is provided at only 68% of first line health facilities, often limited to one day per week. Even less (36%) of first line health facilities provide delivery care. Essential obstetric care service is offered by two hospitals in the district capital.

Process quality

The coverage of antenatal care was 28% for the district (urban 50% vs. rural 24%). Preventive activities such as tetanus vaccination (coverage 51%) and iron supplementation (effective doses 5.2%) are only partially implemented. The national risk catalogue is inflated (47 risk factors) and does not discriminate serious and accepted danger signs from frequent demographic characteristics with low predictive properties. Therefore, it does not promote targeted referral practices. Antenatal care is technically orientated and pays little attention to interpersonal relationship and individual counselling (average counselling time: 1 minute). Out of 41% high risk pregnancies among antenatal attendees, only 15% received a referral advice. This advice was followed in one third of cases, only.

Among 13520 expected deliveries in the district, 1323 took place in hospitals (9.8%). A wide urban-rural disparity is observed (urban 36% vs. rural 4.5%). This is related to greater accessibility for urban women and long distances and high transport costs for women from the rural areas. Caesarean section was performed in only 1.1% of expected deliveries (urban 2.3% vs. rural 0.2%) against a minimum need of 5% according to WHO.

Output and outcome quality

The majority of complicated deliveries occurred outside the health service. Only a small proportion of high risk pregnancies reached the referral hospital (< 5% of previous Caesarean section as well as of pre-eclampsia/eclampsia cases). Thus an important objective of antenatal care was missed. Emergency obstetric admissions were observed rarely (0.3% of expected deliveries) although severe complications in childbirth occur in about 5% of expected deliveries, even among low risk pregnancies. The high stillbirth rate observed in hospital (all deliveries 7%, in Caesarean section cases 14.3%, in breech deliveries 25.8%) indicates deficiencies in hospital-based obstetric care.

Socio-cultural context

Beyond health service factors such as restrictions in access and low quality of care, there are also powerful social and cultural factors that appear to be equally important as reasons for low utilisation of maternity services. These factors are: the traditional perception that pregnancy and childbirth is a process not requiring extra medical care; the courtesy and convenience of home delivery; taboos related to the caste system; the culturally valued women's submission under the elderly; and the perceived illness aetiology influencing the families' health seeking behaviour in pregnancy and childbirth.

Executive summary

The following recommendations are made to improve the maternity services in this district:

- Counselling in antenatal care should be based on women's preferences instead of stereotype risk assignment.

- Accessibility of antenatal and delivery care should be improved by providing services at all first level health facilities.

- Transport mechanisms for obstetric emergencies should be developed on a local level.

- Training and supportive supervision of health workers should be intensified with emphasis on communication and counselling.

- At the national level, maternity care guidelines, including the risk categories, should be critically re-assessed and modified towards a more feasible and user friendly referral practice.

1 Introduction

This study aims to assess antenatal and obstetric care service provided by the modern health service and the communities' views on care during pregnancy and childbirth in Banke district, Nepal. To receive optimum care during pregnancy and childbirth it is necessary to ensure the universally desired outcome of pregnancy, that is to have a healthy mother and a healthy baby. Traditionally, care during pregnancy and childbirth is practised in most societies according to their beliefs and practices. However, some pregnancies end up with tragedies that affect not only the baby and the mother but also the family and the society as well.

Advancement in medical technology and case management, and access to quality health care have contributed to the prevention of most of the maternal and perinatal morbidity and mortality in developed countries (Kaunitz et al. 1984; Rochat, 1981). However, in most developing countries, in spite of high concern and prioritisation of safe motherhood, the maternal and perinatal morbidity and mortality are still unacceptably high (WHO, 1996; WHO, 1994a).

Major killers of pregnant women in developing countries are haemorrhage, hypertensive disorders of pregnancy, puerperal sepsis, unsafe abortion and obstructed labour. At least 15% of all deliveries require skilled obstetric care in the absence of which the mother and or the baby will suffer serious and long-term morbidity and disabilities (WHO, 1994c, p. 1).

Much effort has been directed to identify the causes and to plan effective interventions in order to prevent pregnancy related morbidity and mortality (Maine, 1991; Royston and Armstrong, 1989; Starrs, 1987). Family planning, antenatal care, clean and safe delivery, and essential obstetric care are the four pillars of the safe motherhood programme to prevent death of mothers which occur in the process of pregnancy and childbirth (WHO, 1994c, p. xi).

Antenatal care (ANC) is one of the important health interventions for pregnant women. It has several major functions: promotion of health during pregnancy through advice and educational activities; monitoring the state of health throughout pregnancy in order to detect and deal with problems if and when they occur; and screening, identification and timely referral of women with risk factors (Royston and Armstrong, 1989, p. 157-162).

The World Health Organisation (WHO) has identified specific services that are essential for the care of pregnancy and delivery at the health centre and first referral level in order to save lives of mothers and babies in cases of pregnancy related complications (WHO, 1994b; WHO, 1991a).

To achieve effective interventions, the health service must be organised with a network of community health care workers and first line health services (FLHS) backed up by a properly functioning referral system and a referral level care. Moreover, facilities must be adequately equipped with equipment, drugs, supplies and skilled personnel to provide necessary quality of care, so that the services are accessible and acceptable by the one in need. Otherwise, they are not used by the people for whom they are intended for and also can not provide effective care to the actual users.

Nepal is one of the countries with a high maternal and perinatal mortality rate (maternal mortality ratio 539/100,000 live births, perinatal mortality rate 57/1000 births). Moreover, utilisation of maternity care services is very low in comparison to any other developing country (antenatal care 29% and professional assisted delivery 10%). However, there is little knowledge on the quality of maternity care services and the reasons for low utilisation. This study aims to fill this gap. The ministry of health, His Majesty's government welcome the proposal and granted research permission.

1.1 The purpose of the study

The purpose of this study is to investigate the existing maternal health care services in Banke district, Nepal.

1.1.1 The study questions

1. How good is the quality of care provided by the modern health services regarding pregnancy and childbirth?

2. How does the community perceive the care provided by modern health service and what are the patterns of the community's health-seeking behaviour regarding pregnancy and childbirth?

1.1.2 The study objectives

By investigating and coming forward with conclusions and recommendations, this study aims to contribute to the amelioration of the existing maternity care services.

General objective:

To assess antenatal and obstetric care services in Banke District, Nepal.

Specific objectives:

1. To analyse the existing health services in terms of accessibility and availability.

2. To determine the actual utilisation of antenatal and obstetric care services with regards to specific providers and levels of care.

3. To analyse health services performance with emphasis on high risk pregnancies and deliveries.

4. To identify bottlenecks in the pathway from screening to appropriate management.

5. To analyse the health seeking behaviour of the community and the perception of modern health care with regards to pregnancy and childbirth.

've
2 Literature Review

2.1 Introduction

This study describes the situation of antenatal and obstetric care services in Banke district, Nepal with emphasis on assessment of actual utilisation with the determinants of utilisation and the quality of services delivered. Community perspectives on care regarding pregnancy and childbirth were included for a comprehensive understanding of the situation and to be able to draw concrete recommendations.

The literature review will be divided into three parts. Firstly, the country background of this study will be presented. The second part will address the general overview of the safe motherhood programmes as recommended in the international literature and thirdly, literature on the assessment of antenatal and obstetric care service including methodological aspects will be presented.

2.2 Nepal: the country background

2.2.1 Geography and demography

Nepal is a landlocked country situated on the southern slope of the Himalayas between 26° 22' and 30° 27' north latitudes and 80° 15' and 88° 19' east longitudes, an irregular rectangle shape, extending from east to west. The total land area is 147,181 sq. km, covering three different ecological regions namely *terai* (plain), hilly and mountainous regions. Administratively the country is divided as eastern, central, western, mid-western, and far-western development regions.

The total population counts 18.5 million in the 1991 census. 9% of the population live in urban area. The estimated population growth rate was 2.1% per year and mean age at marriage was 21.4 for male and 18.2 for female in 1991. The estimated population projection for 1996/97 was 22 million. Its population is relatively young with 40% of the population under 15.

Some national health indicators are as follows. Crude birth rate 41.5/1000 population; crude death rate 14.85/1000 population; total fertility rate 4.6 births per women; infant mortality rate 83/1000 live birth (LB); perinatal mortality rate (PNMR) 57/1000 total births; maternal mortality ratio (MMR) 539/100,000 LB accounting for 27% of all deaths of reproductive age women. 29% currently married women use a family planning method. Life expectancy was 55 years for males and 53.5 years for females in 1991 (Pradhan et al. 1996).

2.2.2 Politics, economy and society

Nepal is a country with a monarchy and parliamentary democracy. Since 1991, His Majesty's Government (HMG) is elected democratically.

The gross national product (GNP) per capita was US$ 200 in 1995. 48% of the gross domestic products come from the service sector, 42% from agricultural sector and 10% from manufacturing sector. 53% of the population live below the poverty line (World Bank, 1997; Pradhan et al. 1996).

The main crops of the country are rice, wheat and corn. The majority of the population live with subsistence farming especially in rural area. 90% of employed women are engaged in the agricultural sector (Pradhan et al. 1996).

Nepal is a multi-ethnic and multi-lingual society with about 60 ethnic groups and sub-groups, and 20 different languages and dialects, originating from Indo-Aryans (80%) and Tibetan-Burmese (17%). The official language is *Nepali*. Each community has its own rules and regulations concerning women's mobility, marriage options, access to resources and social status.

Nepali women are lag far behind men in many aspects of development indicators such as literacy rate, property possession and employment. However, they are taking the major economic responsibility within the family. Health care decisions for women are mainly made by senior members of the family, mainly mothers-in-law (Steinmann and Ramji, 1996). Their ability to have a child (especially son) is the road for their security (Acharya, 1997). The sufferings related to pregnancy and childbirth and unacceptably high maternal deaths still continue and are among the highest in developing countries (Pradhan et al. 1996; Smith et al. 1996).

2.2.3 The health care system

The health care system of Nepal includes public sector, private sector, non-governmental organisation sector and traditional medicine sector. The national health spending is 6% of GNP in 1996/97.

The National Health Policy (1991) focuses on increasing the accessibility of the rural population to primary health care services. Service delivery focuses on the community with training of female community health volunteer (FCHV) (1:150 population in mountainous region, 1:250 population in hilly region and 1:400 population in Teria region) and training of traditional birth attendants (TBA)

(1:500 for mountainous, 1:1000 for hilly and 1:1500 for Teria region). This community level health care delivery is backed up by a network of first line health services (FLHS) including one sub-health post (SHP) or health post (HP) in one village development committee and one primary health centre (PHC) in each electoral constituency with no hospital. This in turn should be backed up by a referral mechanism and specialised services at the referral level.

In the public sector, health care delivery is executed through the department of health services under the Ministry of Health (MoH). There are 5 regional health service directorates, 75 district health offices with a networks of primary health care services including 205 PHC, 611 HP, and 3199 SHP in the village level. About 20 hospitals are able to provide essential obstetric care (EOC).

The private sector includes a number of nursing homes and hospitals providing all levels of health care and doctors' private clinics in urban areas. The traditional medical sector includes Ayurveda, Homeopathy, Unani, Naturopathy and Tibetan medicine. Faith healing is also widely practised (Ramji, 1997).

2.2.4 Nepal's safe motherhood policy and programme

Nepal's national safe motherhood programme was designed in response to international call for safe motherhood. The policy is directed not only to the health services but also to the family and community as well as empowerment of women. The main strategies of the safe motherhood programme focus on improving the quality and the coverage of maternal health care services to all women at the three main levels of the districts:

- At a family or community level by encouraging appropriate decision-making for the care of pregnant women through appropriate information, organising community support services, and strengthening delivery of maternity services by trained TBA and FCHV.
- At FLHS level by delivering maternity care services by adequately trained and skilled staff.
- At hospital level by upgrading their physical infra-structure and strengthening their capability to provide essential obstetric care (UNICEF and MoH, 1996).

The safe motherhood programme was implemented in 10 districts as a first phase and a national maternity care guideline was developed as a tool for implementing the safe motherhood programme in 1996 (UNICEF and MoH,

1996). The target for safe motherhood in the 9th National Health Plan (1997/2002), was to reduce maternal mortality by 20% (400 per 100,000 LB) at the end of the year 2002.

The national antenatal risk catalogue

The national risk catalogue for antenatal care is comparable with internationally agreed risk catalogues except for some modification according to the population status. The following are categorised as high risk pregnancy in the national maternity care guideline of Nepal. Action to be taken should be considered according to individual status (UNICEF and MoH, 1996).

General:
- age at first pregnancy 19 years and below or 35 years and above,
- height below, 148cm (4' 10''),
- parity 4th and above,
- unmarried mother.

Events during previous pregnancies:
- repeated pregnancy loss (3 or more consecutive abortion),
- previous intrauterine death,
- previous premature delivery,
- previous neonatal death, congenital defect in new-born,
- history of sub-fertility,
- history of post-partum haemorrhage (PPH) and/or retained placenta,
- prolonged labour and assisted deliveries.

Medical disorder:
- anaemia,
- hypertensive disorder,
- diabetes,
- renal disease,
- jaundice,
- tuberculosis,
- cardio-vascular disease,
- endocrine disorder,
- severe malnutrition or obesity.

History of smoking, alcohol or drug consumption.

Surgical conditions:
- previous Caesarean section (CS),

Literature review

- pelvic floor repair, vesico-vaginal fistula repair,
- hysterotomy, myomectomy,
- tubal reconstruction surgery,
- pregnancy with fibroid, ovarian cyst and carcinoma cervix.

Events during present pregnancy:
- pre-eclampsia and eclampsia (blood pressure (BP) >= 140/90 mmHg),
- bleeding during pregnancy,
- mal-presentation,
- cephalo-pelvic disproportion,
- multiple pregnancy,
- polyhydramnios, oligohydramnios,
- small for dates,
- post-maturity,
- rhesus negative,
- premature rupture of membrane,
- premature labour,
- infection including sexually transmitted diseases (STD) and
- Human Immuno-deficiency Virus (HIV).

Miscellaneous:
- no ANC or less than 2 visits,
- past history of blood transfusion,
- time since last delivery <2 or > 10 years,
- weight gain in pregnancy < 7 kg or > 14 kg,
- past history of babies > 4000kg, and
- congenital genital tract anomalies.

2.3 The global safe motherhood programme

2.3.1 The concept and goal of the global safe motherhood initiative

The concept of safe motherhood initiative stems from the high discrepancy of maternal mortality between developed and developing countries and the realisation that most of these deaths can be prevented by publicising and attacking the problems. A global target "to reduce maternal deaths by 50% by the year 2000" was set by the international safe motherhood conference at Nairobi in 1987 (Starrs, 1987, p. 8).

Safe motherhood is defined by Feuerstein 1993, as "creating the circumstances within which a woman is enabled to choose whether she will become pregnant, and if she does, ensuring she receives care for prevention and treatment of pregnancy complications, has access to trained birth assistance, has access to emergency obstetric care if she needs it, and care after birth, so that she can avoid death or disability from complications of pregnancy and childbirth" (Feuerstein, 1993, p. 2).

Starting with avoiding unplanned and undesired pregnancy (family planning), promotion of health of the pregnant women, planning and implementation of clean and safe delivery, prevention and management of complications arising during pregnancy and delivery together with a functioning referral system, and post-natal care were the different strategies of the safe motherhood programme.

2.3.2 The history of safe motherhood programmes

The practice of antenatal care and care during childbirth by modern health services had started during the early seventeenth century in Europe. Maternal mortality rate among members of the ruling houses of Europe was about 2000 per 100,000 LB during the 16th, 17th, and 18th centuries and 1470 per 100,000 LB during the last half of 19th century (Peller, 1965 cited by Rochat, 1981). It started to decline with the introduction of compulsory obstetric care by trained midwives in Sweden and other parts of Europe from early and late 19th century respectively. Consequently, it declined to the present level of 7 per 100,000 LB in Sweden and 36 per 100,000 LB in Europe with the help of improved service organisation, modern technology, education and the improvement in socio-economic conditions.

In developing countries, maternal health care has been a neglected area throughout history leading to an unacceptably high discrepancy of maternal mortality between developed and developing world. It was not the priority for policy and health planners until early 1970s. Under the Primary Health Care concept of Alma-Ata, maternal and child health care was regarded as a high priority in the strategy for "Health For All by the Year 2000". However, the maternal mortality in many developing countries is still as high as the maternal mortality rate in the previous century Europe.

The importance of maternal health was highlighted in particular during the United Nation Women's Decade (1975-84) and more specifically in a 1985 article entitled "Maternal mortality- A neglected tragedy: Where is M in MCH?" by Rosenfield and Maine (1985). In 1987, a 'Safe Motherhood Initiative' was called at the Nairobi International Safe Motherhood Conference to prevent maternal deaths (Starrs, 1987).

Many strategies have been introduced to improve maternal and child health care (MCH) in various countries by various agencies. The basic objectives of maternal health care aimed at reducing the numbers of high risk and unwanted pregnancies, reducing obstetric complications, and reducing case fatality rates in women with complications. To meet these objectives a practical guide for implementing safe motherhood was developed by WHO (WHO, 1994b & c).

In spite of all these efforts to improve maternal health condition and after a decade of Safe motherhood Initiatives, maternal suffering and mortality is still unacceptably high in many developing countries with the global maternal mortality ratio (MMR) at 480 per 100,000 LB (approximately 585,000 women per year). During World Health Day, 1998, safe motherhood activities were relaunched with the slogan "pregnancy is special - let's make it safe".

2.3.3 The criticisms of safe motherhood programmes
2.3.3.1 Antenatal care

The objective of antenatal care is to ensure safe pregnancy and delivery for all pregnant women. There is general agreement that the model of antenatal care is good: "The concept of risk approach in ANC is generally recognised as a very good model of preventive health care" (Villar and Bergsjo, 1997). A series of health examinations aiming to promote health and to prevent and manage adverse outcome of pregnancy and delivery should make the health service to be able to achieve the objectives of antenatal care.

However, questions have been asked about the possible impact of antenatal care on maternal mortality as early as 1932 by Browne & Aberd (cited by McDonagh 1996). The main reasons for failures seem to be due to failure to recognise many problems and danger signs during pregnancy and childbirth together with the low predictive value of most risk screening procedures and further failure to implement proper management of identified risk (McDonagh, 1996; Winikoff, 1995; Rooney, 1992; Hall et al. 1980).

One fundamental problem is that risk screening has such a low predictive value that many women are referred unnecessarily, causing undue stress and cost to the family as well as to the health system. This is mainly due to a lack of controlled trials to prove the effectiveness of procedures used in antenatal care and their effect on maternal mortality (Rooney, 1992; Lindmark and Cnattingius, 1991; Hall et al. 1980).

Moreover, low specificity has also been remarked as many women identified as non-risk develop complications during pregnancy and childbirth. In the USA, among low risk women who delivered at birth centres, 7.9% developed serious complications to mother and/or baby during and immediately after delivery. 2.4% needed emergency operations (Rooks et al. 1989). McDonagh (1996) further emphasises that antenatal care is a preventive care that is voluntary in nature. As the service could cover only those who come voluntarily, it misses the ones who are in most need of care.

In spite of criticising the effectiveness of antenatal care, there are many activities that are effective in detecting, treating or preventing conditions in pregnancy that may lead to serious morbidity and mortality such as anaemia, infections, hypertensive disorder of pregnancy and neonatal tetanus (Rooney, 1992, p. 35).

To be effective, antenatal care should be a part of health care system backed up by good local obstetric care at community level, essential obstetric care at referral level and a functioning referral system. The importance of these have been highlighted by Rooney (1992) by stating "even high quality antenatal care cannot be a substitute for adequate emergency access to obstetric service" (Rooney, 1992, p. 12).

2.3.3.2 Obstetric care

The absence of clean and safe delivery together with inaccessibility of emergency obstetric care services have been seen as one of the most important reasons for maternal deaths (Thaddeus and Maine, 1994; Royston and Armstrong, 1989; Gadalla et al. 1987; Kaunitz et al. 1984). The importance of this has been repeatedly advocated to reduce maternal mortality (McCarthy, 1997; WHO, 1991a; Kwast, 1989; Rosenfield and Maine, 1985).

Many programmes have been launched to improve obstetric care services in different parts of the world namely training programmes for traditional birth attendants, strengthening capability of FLHS in tackling obstetric emergencies (essential obstetric care at FLHS level), mobilisation of community and emer-

Literature review 13

gency transport, and strengthening district hospital (essential obstetric care at referral level).

TBA training programmes were seen as successful for overcoming cultural barriers for using assisted delivery, conveying knowledge and for provision of clean delivery (Dehne et al. 1995; Rizvi, 1994; Greenwood et al. 1987, Bhatia, 1981). However, many other studies show failure of these programmes due to non-use of their service (Bhatia and Cleland, 1995; Nougtara et al. 1989). The reasons identified were mainly deficits in the health system like lack of supervision and support, and the presence of quality consciousness of the community (Campbell and Sham, 1995; Nougtara et al. 1989). Maine (1991) calculates TBA training programmes as the most expensive programmes in terms of preventing maternal deaths. Others also support this finding (McCarthy, 1997).

There are many studies that show effectiveness of upgrading midwifery skills of FLHS workers in preventing maternal mortality (Maine et al. 1996; Bergström and da Luz Vaz, 1992; Taylor et al. 1992). The experiences from "the prevention of maternal mortality network" (PMMN) in western Africa show that many maternal deaths could be prevented with simple and cheap programmes using community resources and delegating responsibilities to midwives backed up with referral level care (Maine, 1997). However, sustainability of these programmes is questionable. Rooney (1992) stresses the difficulty in sustaining these programme by stating "effective treatment should be provided at the most peripheral or local level at which it is safe to do so, bearing in mind the necessity to train and motivate staff and the need to maintain their expertise".

Experience has shown that the success of such programmes often depends on community involvement. Maine (1991) suggests community mobilisation could facilitate access to emergency obstetric care in case of complications. This has been proven in utilisation of maternal health care services in Nigeria (Okafor, 1991). In the PMMN group, communities were effectively mobilised for emergency transport, leading to an increased number of obstetric complications admitted to hospital. Emergency transport has reduced the case fatality rate of obstetric complications by 50% in one study group (Samai and Sengeh, 1997).

WHO (1991a) advocates the essential elements of obstetric care at first referral level hospital in order to treat obstetric complications. The elements include: (1) surgical obstetrics, (2) anaesthesia, (3) medical treatment, (4) replacement of blood, (5) manual procedure and continuous monitoring of labour, (6) management of women at high risk, (7) family planning support, and (8) neonatal special care.

However, many hospitals in developing countries are deficient in quality and capability to implement essential obstetric care (Jafarey and Korejo, 1993; Walker et al. 1986). This is exaggerated by accessibility problems (Dujardin et al. 1995; Thaddeus and Maine, 1994), leading to a condition where mothers are dying of the preventable causes. Maine (1991) discusses the reasons behind the difficulties of focusing on strengthening hospitals to provide EOC. One is that the current emphasis is on primary health care. Secondly, people assume that most obstetric complications can be prevented and another impeding factor is the cost of improving obstetric care at hospital level.

2.3.3.3 Post-natal care and family planning

The occurrence of the highest number of maternal deaths (60%) during the post-partum period leads to concern of many health planners about the importance of post-natal care. Dissemination of information about danger signs and symptom in this period and the importance of early referral to hospital is crucial in this period. However, in spite of high coverage for antenatal care, coverage of post-natal check up is lower in many parts of the world. Post-natal check up was attended by one out of five women who attend ANC in India and was almost non-existent in Tanzania (Oyeledun, 1997; Bhatia and Cleland, 1995). Moreover, there is no counselling of mothers on danger signs during their post-natal check up, leaving maternal mortality still highest in this period.

The effect of family planning on maternal mortality by reducing unnecessary pregnancies (too early, too many, too frequent and too late) has been stressed by many authors (WHO, 1994; Maine, 1991; Royston and Armstrong, 1989; Gadalla et al. 1987). However, in spite of high concern and implementation of family planning programmes in various countries, many couples still have unmet needs concerning family planning.

2.4 Assessing antenatal and obstetric care services

Pregnancy and childbirth are normal physiological processes with favourable outcome in most cases. However, no pregnancy and childbirth are without risks to the mother and/or the baby. Traditionally, recognising these risks, many cultures care for pregnant women with different beliefs and practices to prevent deaths and suffering related to pregnancy and childbirth. With advance in technology and health service organisation and better socio-economic conditions, maternal mortality has been declining to the present level of 11 & 36 per 100,000 LB in USA and Europe.

In developing countries, maternal mortality ratio remains very high, 480 per 100,000 LB (WHO 1996). A number of researches were carried out to find out reasons for this and to improve service delivery in maternal health care to prevent sufferings and deaths related to pregnancy and childbirth. Low quality of maternal health care services was recognised along with accessibility problems. Furthermore, there is a general agreement that interventions to improve health of mothers and babies can only be achieved by approaches that promote equity in access and quality of care.

2.4.1 Definition of quality and methodological issues in quality assessment

In the late 80s, quality of care has become a focal interest for many health planners as accessibility alone does not guarantee the utilisation of services. Moreover, willingness to pay for services depends on perceived service quality as well as community's perception on quality of care (Sauerborn et al. 1989; Annis, 1981). The reason behind the previous low interest in quality issues was a perceived priority of quantity (mainly coverage and utilisation) over quality. Additionally, the perception existed that improving quality requires increasing inputs, thus being costly and not affordable for many countries (Sauerborn and Reerink, 1996; Razum, 1994).

Roemer & Montoya-Aguilar (1988), define quality of health care as "the degree to which the resource for health care or the services included in health care correspond to specific standard. Those standards, if applied, are generally expected to lead to desired results ----------------- to improve the outcome or effectiveness of programme".

Donabedian defines quality as "quality is proportionate to the attainment of achievable improvement in health". His approach to quality assessment is to examine the characteristics of the setting in which care is provided (structure), to examine the attributes of the process of care itself (process), and to examine the effects of care on the health and welfare of individuals or populations (output/outcome). Moreover, assessment of patient satisfaction should also be included in quality assessment as it reflects the patient judgement on all aspects of care (Donabedian, 1988a & 1988b). The main purpose of quality assessment is to identify strengths of the programme and areas of weakness within a programme that call for strengthening (Roemer & Montoya-Aguilar, 1988, Donabedian, 1988b).

Maternal mortality and perinatal mortality rate have been used as indicators to assess maternal health care programmes. Another indicator recently used in assessment of health service is user satisfaction. The use of mortality rate for measuring programme success has been questioned. The reasons are that assessment of maternal mortality is neither easy nor cheap nor complete and mortality rate is influenced by many other factors (Graham and Airey, 1987). For example, in Matlab, Bangladesh, an intervention trial was implemented to find out the effectiveness of extensive midwife's service with emergency referral backed up by a fully equipped hospital that can deal with emergency obstetric conditions. The programme claimed a decline in maternal mortality in the intervention areas after three years of implementation (Maine et al. 1996). However, a decline in maternal mortality was also experienced by the areas without programme implementation, calling for caution in the interpretation of programme success by one outcome indicator (Ronsman, 1997). Others also suggested that maternal mortality rate should be used as an evidence that prompts and motivates the assessment of the health service in the search for conditions that can be improved (Donabedian, 1988b) and as for making policy and planning (Campbell et al. 1997).

Recently, perinatal mortality rate has been proposed as a proxy indicator for service quality of maternal health care programmes (Mancey-Jones and Brugha, 1997). However, its use has been questioned as causes of perinatal and maternal mortality are not necessarily similar in many cases (Akalin et al. 1997).

Assessment of structural availability is rather simple and studies were conducted to identify weaknesses in this area that contribute to lack of quality health care. Garner et al. (1990) present a method for structural assessment of health facilities in rural Papua New Guinea, using a checklist based on the presence or absence of certain equipment and drugs. Although structural quality is a prerequisite for a system to provide care (Gilson et al. 1995), it is rather a blunt instrument to assess quality. As Bobadilla (1992) points out: "Lack of essential resources can reasonably lead to lower effectiveness, but availability does not necessarily guarantee good performance or satisfactory outcome".

As maternal mortality is difficult to measure as well as governed by many factors, and structural quality does not guarantee for good quality of care, many authors suggest to use a wide variety of service delivery process indicators (Campbell et al. 1997; Razum, 1994). Tinker and Koblinsky (1993) state that: "The programme goal may be to reduce maternal mortality, emphasis should be given to measuring the processes and factors that are known to reduce maternal mortality". Process evaluation determines whether a programme is being implemented as planned (Klein 1983, cited by Razum 1994).

There are different variables used to assess the structural and process quality such as availability, accessibility, utilisation and service quality (adherence to standard). However, a multi-dimensional approach combining all four variables with user satisfaction is appropriate to assess quality of health care programme especially where utilisation is low (Razum 1994, p. 15-23). Peters & Becker (1991) present a multi-dimensional approach by using several methods including a facility checklist, revision of medical records, structured observation of immunisation process and interviewing health workers for their knowledge for assessing quality of care in key child survival activities in the Philippines. The observational method was recommended as a simple and useful method that gives information about provider-patient interaction.

Assessing quality of health care services is incomplete without assessing the perception of community on health services and health care itself which influence acceptability and utilisation of health services (Razum, 1994; Donabedian, 1990).

The following sections will emphasise literature on assessment of quality of antenatal and obstetric care services from both the service point of view (2.4.2) and the community point of view (2.4.3).

2.4.2 Assessment of quality of antenatal and obstetric care service

There are many studies assessing quality of antenatal and obstetric care services focusing on availability, accessibility, coverage, service quality (technical and interpersonal process) and users' satisfaction as well as its impact on maternal and perinatal mortality. Although a more-dimensional approach covering all variables is more desirable for assessing the service quality, the literature review will cover the variables separately for easier understanding.

2.4.2.1 Availability

To provide effective health care, the facility should be available and the health care environment should be convenient for the provider as well as the client. Availability is the ratio between the population and health personnel or facilities offering the service. Indicators showing availability of facilities and staff are used as one of the basic health care indicator for a given country and emphasis has been made on per capita availability at different levels of care to ensure equity in health care delivery. Moreover, a guideline for essential equipment, drugs and consumable needed for different levels of health facilities was prepared by WHO as well as by national health planners (UNICEF and MoH, 1996; WHO, 1994b; WHO, 1994c).

In response to this, many studies have focused on the assessment of structural quality: availability of facility, staff and of essential equipment, drugs and consumable in many areas, especially in rural areas. Availability of equipment, drugs and supplies was assessed by a checklist, availability at the time of assessment or by checking availability during a number of months in a year (Kielmann et al. 1991; Garner et al. 1990).

Although availability does not necessarily guarantee the provision of quality care, studies showed that lack of facility, staff, equipment, drugs and supplies were associated with increased case fatality rate of obstetric complications (PMMN, 1992). Moreover, these factors also influence users' perception on health services. Absence of equipment, drugs and supplies as well as the purchasing cost was perceived as barriers to use these services and causing delay in seeking care (Okafor and Rizzuto, 1994; PMMN, 1992).

2.4.2.2 Accessibility

Equity, that is fairness in the distribution of care, is the foundation on which the four pillars of safe motherhood namely family planning, antenatal care, clean and safe delivery, and essential obstetric care, are based (WHO, 1994c). Equity is seen as one feature of quality care (Donabedian, 1990). Inequity in health care due to unequal access (including geographical, financial and socio-cultural accessibility) in developing countries is one of the important factors that leads to most of maternal deaths and sufferings (Thaddeus and Maine, 1994). Access to health care is mainly assessed in relation to utilisation of health services by potential users and their health care outcome. Although the effects of accessibility variables on utilisation of health services are interrelated they will be presented separately.

Geographical accessibility

Assessment of geographical accessibility (equitable distribution) was mainly done with assessing utilisation of health services in relation to distance between potential patient and the nearest health facility and its impacts on health outcome. Thaddeus & Maine (1994) discuss how distance could influence utilisation: long distance can be an actual obstacle to reach a health facility, and a disincentive to trying to seek care. Difficulties in transportation and poor roads in many parts of the world add this obstacle.

Review of hospitals and health centres records revealed that there is a linear relationship between utilisation and distance, the proportion of users declines as the radius increase. For example, per capita utilisation decline with distance in Nigeria (Stock, 1983), in rural Tanzania (Jahn et al. 1998), and in rural Zaire, most major obstetric interventions are performed on women from within 60 Km distance (van Lerberghe et al. 1988).

Individual interviews with service users and/or non-users revealed that distance plays an important disincentive role in deterring use of service. It was shown for normal delivery (Voorhoeve et al. 1984), antenatal referral compliance (Dujardin et al. 1995), for emergency obstetric cases (PMMN, 1992), and in other illnesses (Csete, 1993). One of the reasons for higher mortality rate among rural population is geographical inaccessibility (Greenwood et al. 1987; Lamb et al. 1984).

Although unequal distribution of health services is blamed as a reason for non-use of services, the presence of health services does not necessarily guarantee for quality care as well as utilisation of these services (Annis, 1981). Distance was less important than level of service in utilisation of maternal health care services in Burkina Faso (Nougtara et al. 1989). Moreover, quality also implies acceptability which is shaped by many other factors such as cost and effectiveness (Donabedian, 1990).

Financial accessibility

Another factor that is important in delivery of equitable health care is the cost of care born by the clients. In many developing countries, economic crisis together with the introduction of co-financing in health care including service fees, cost for medications and materials, cost for transport, and opportunity cost deter utilisation of health services as well as delay decision to seek care (Thaddeus and Maine, 1994).

The effect of financial inaccessibility on utilisation of health services is mainly assessed by individual interviews to evaluate the users' perception on financial accessibility or by reviewing health services registers. Household surveys are useful to find the relationship between health service utilisation and the user's socio-economic characteristics (Bhatia and Cleland, 1995; Obermeyer, 1993; Egunjobi, 1983).

Although cost was not the most important deterring factors for utilisation of health services in some studies (Kloos et al. 1987; Egunjobi, 1983), increases in maternal health care utilisation were found with higher government spending on health (Obermeyer, 1993), with increase in family income in Columbia (Montoya-Aguilar and Marin-Lira, 1986), and use of private services with higher income in India (Bhatia and Cleland, 1995).

Socio-cultural accessibility

The importance of a socially and culturally acceptable health care system in the delivery of modern health care can not be over emphasised. It is a prerequisite for utilisation of health service. Assessment is done by individual and focus group interviews with health service users and non-users (Maier et al. 1994, p. 1-6).

Social distance between health care provider and the potential users was perceived as an important barrier for utilisation of services among highlander Ecuador (Finerman, 1983). The same barrier as well as barriers due to languages and bad staff attitudes were experienced for utilisation of emergency obstetric care services in western Africa (PMMN, 1992). Feeling as a stranger and uneasiness in the hospital surrounding were mentioned by rural women of southern Tanzania as a barrier to seek care at referral level (Kowalewski et al. 1998). Culturally valued traditions and practices not accommodated in hospital regulations was also perceived as a barrier for using hospital delivery care services. For example, episiotomy was frequently done during hospital deliveries whereas traditionally it is considered as loss of women-hood in western Africa (Ityavyar, 1984).

2.4.2.3 Coverage (Utilisation)

Coverage is perceived as one indicator that is related to outcome of health care and it has been recommended for assessing service quality of health service (Tinker and Koblinsky, 1993; WHO, 1994a; Campbell et al. 1997).Coverage is defined as "The ratio of population served with an activity to the population in need of the activity" (Montoya-Aguilar, 1994). The concept of coverage is concerned with a target population and the actual use of health services by the population. It is influenced by availability, accessibility and acceptability of health service for a given population.

Tinker & Koblinsky (1993) suggest a wide range of process indicators for assessing maternal health programmes such as coverage of antenatal care, timeliness of antenatal care, coverage of TT immunisation, coverage of anaemia prophylactics, referral rate and referral compliance, coverage of delivery and post-partum care, and % of women with low socio-economic status using maternity care service.

Coverage related to antenatal and delivery care were obtained from household surveys as in demographic and health survey data or review of registers from hospitals and health centres. Coverage stratified with socio-economic status and distance from the health facilities gives the utilisation pattern and accessibility of health care by different social strata. Moreover, coverage of different obstetric complications by a hospital shows the accessibility as well as the quality of health care process (Campbell et al. 1997). Recently, the coverage of major obstetric interventions in absolute maternal indications was advocated to monitor the unmet obstetric need (UON) of a district (Belghiti et al. 1998).

WHO has produced estimated data on coverage of antenatal and maternity care for different countries. However, coverage related to post-partum care was found to be scarce (WHO, 1997; Bhatia and Cleland, 1995). The latest demographic and health survey in Nepal showed that 29.3% of women received antenatal care service from trained health workers at least once during their last pregnancy and 10.1% delivered with trained attendants. Post natal care was received by 13% within 24 hours of delivery in that survey. Coverage of antenatal care was highest among younger age group and among women with at least primary education (Pradhan et al. 1996).

In a recent study from India, 95% of women have at least one antenatal care visit, 39% delivered with trained assistants and 20% had post-partum check up in their last pregnancy and delivery (Bhatia and Cleland, 1995). Similarly, although 100% antenatal care coverage was observed in rural Tanzania, delivery care coverage was 35% and post-partum care was "almost non-existing" (Oyeledun, 1997). In rural Burkina Faso, 31% of mothers interviewed had received antenatal care and 32% had delivery with a trained assistant in their last pregnancy. 60% of women delivered with an old woman from the village (Nougtara et al. 1989).

2.4.2.4 Performance of health services (service quality)

Provision of good quality health care is necessary to achieve desired outcomes. Lack of quality in maternal health care services has been frequently blamed as the cause of many maternal deaths as well as the reason for non-use of health services. It was also found that when a user has access to different alternatives of health care, perceived high quality of care overcome distance barriers (Nougtara et al. 1989; Stock, 1983) and financial barriers (Kloos et al. 1987).

Service quality is defined as "What is actually performed with a relevant standard" (Montoya-Aguilar, 1994). With antenatal and obstetric care, it implies adherence to timing and content of procedures and ability to follow the risk approach in antenatal care. The importance of assessing service quality (process quality), technical process as well as interpersonal process, has been emphasised by many authors (Adeyi and Morrow, 1996; Montoya-Aguilar, 1994; Razum, 1994; Peters and Becker, 1991; Donabedian, 1988a).

In assessment of quality, difficulties exist in verifying "standard" which is defined as "a precise, numerical goodness with regard to each of the phenomena (parameter) under study" (Donabedian, 1981). Bobadilla (1992) presents possible ways to define standard namely theoretical, best possible and best achievable. A system of maximum obtainable score, that is 100%, was used in the assessment of antenatal consultation processes in rural India. Observation of antenatal consultation was done with the help of a standardised checklist. The mean score of each component of antenatal care was expressed as a percentage of maximum obtainable score (Srinivasa et al. 1982). Implicit judgement and audit scoring of records done by a third party were used in Kenya to assess the quality of antenatal care process (Malone, 1980).

Literature review

Many studies applied observation of the care process. Review of recent records was recommended over performance observation and review of old records from a study assessing EOC (Adeyi and Morrow, 1996). Studies using situational analysis look for the quality of health care activities to determine the extent to which the activity meets the intended outcome in obstetric care services (PMMN, 1995). Audit of maternal deaths in order to find whether the death could have been avoidable was done for assessing the quality of maternity care services (Hoestermann et al. 1996; Walker et al. 1986). Audit of "near-missed" cases was recently advocated to assess the quality of hospital obstetric care services (Campbell et al. 1997).

Inadequate quality of care in many institutions was revealed in extensive literature reviews regarding antenatal care (Villar and Bergsjo, 1997; McDonagh, 1996; Rooney, 1992) and essential obstetric care (Thaddeus and Maine, 1994). Thaddeus and Maine (1994) extensively discuss how low quality could cause delay in health care seeking, which is detrimental to the health of both the mother and the baby especially in cases of obstetric emergency. From the client's perspective, quality encompasses the effectiveness of treatment as well as availability of supplies and interpersonal relationship between health workers and client. They pointed out that the potential users may delay the decision to seek care until the seriousness of the condition makes necessary overcoming all the barriers. In west Africa, the PMMN group found that communities are aware of deficiencies in the services. Lack of trained staff, delay in attendance by staff even in emergency cases and communication problems were perceived as barriers to seek care (PMMN, 1992). Situational analysis of maternal health care in Sudan revealed that health workers of all level in Ministry of Health are limited in their ability to prevent, diagnose and manage complication during pregnancy and labour (Campbell and Sham, 1995).

Some hospital-based studies tried to discriminate maternal deaths in hospitals into avoidable and unavoidable deaths. Many of them were identified as entirely or probably avoidable. In Gambia, 51% of all maternal deaths at the referral hospital could have been avoided by proper and adequate care at the hospital (Hoestermann et al. 1996). In Jamaica, it was found out that 68% of maternal deaths in hospital are associated with avoidable factors in the health service (Walker et al. 1986). In Pakistan, one of the reason for delay in seeking care in 'mothers brought dead cases' was inadequate and inefficient health services while most mothers lived within 6-8 Km distance from the hospital (Jafarey and Korejo, 1993).

2.4.2.5 User satisfaction

The quality of a health care system is also reflected in its ability to satisfy patients. Patient satisfaction is the additional outcome of health care process and considered as one dimension of quality assessment (Razum, 1994). Satisfaction or dissatisfaction reflects the patient's judgement on all aspects of health care including availability, accessibility, the service quality and the outcome of care. It also modifies their acceptability of health care (Donabedian, 1988b).

In his paper of "quality assessment and assurance", Donabedian discusses the pivotal role played by user satisfaction on the health care as satisfied patients are more likely to co-operate in the implementation of care (Donabedian, 1988b). Thaddeus and Maine (1994) discuss that user satisfaction/dissatisfaction can be stemming from the outcome of health care (e.g. effectiveness of treatment) as well as from the service received (e.g. availability of supplies, hospital procedure, staff attitude). They also indicate that when patients are dissatisfied with services such as procedures performed, staff attitude and long waiting time, this tends to affect their decision to seek care.

Although the importance of user satisfaction in quality health care has been emphasised by many authors, few studies have assessed user satisfaction in assessment of health care quality. Reasons were technically orientated providers, the sensitive nature of assessing user satisfaction, and the unavailability of information about interpersonal processes in records and registers (Donabedian, 1988b).

Some studies used the impact of service organisation and waiting time on acceptability of services offered. Long waiting time and short contact time (mean 69 min, 11.8 min) together with inappropriate service hours and fragmentation of services were seen as factor that hinders acceptability of MCH services in rural Burkina Faso. The importance of time spent by mothers at services, especially when women are involving in agricultural production and caring of family was highlighted by stating that "not true to call the services free of cost" (Sauerborn et al. 1989). Observing inappropriate service hours and fragmentation of services in urban Nigeria, for economically active women, Bamisaiye (1986) also recommends to reform organisation of service to improve the coverage of MCH services. Long waiting time was listed as the least liked feature of the service by the clients interviewed in rural Tanzania (Oyeledun, 1997).

Literature review 25

2.4.3 Assessment of community perspectives on care during pregnancy and childbirth

The health system encompasses providers as well as users. The users must make use of the health care provided to fulfil the objectives of the health system. When the services are not used to their full potential, it becomes important to find out the community's perspectives on health care as well as on available health services.

There are studies and literature reviews that explore barriers behind utilisation of antenatal and obstetric care services in many countries and in different cultures. Although the reasons for non-use of health services were generally identified as health service factors, socio-cultural factor and individual factors, community perspectives on modern health services differ from community to community and culture to culture. (Campanella et al. 1993; PMMN, 1992; Royston and Armstrong, 1989).

There are few studies exploring the reasons behind utilisation and non-utilisation of maternal health care services as well as community perspectives on modern health services in Nepal. Qualitative research becomes important when the researcher does not have pre-defined ideas about the situation he/she explored (Maier et al. 1994, p. 1-6). Qualitative research methodology using focus group discussions and key-informants' interviews were applied to explore this area in maternal health care.

Focus group discussion allows the researcher access to a large body of information in a relatively short time. It is not representative, but has self-correcting mechanism. Key-informants are people who have special position in the community and are looked upon as representatives of the opinions and experiences of a whole group. They can provide valuable and independent information about the whole community, or a group of people in a fairly short period of time (Maier et al. 1994, p. 36-43).

2.4.3.1 Beliefs and practices of community regarding pregnancy and childbirth

Although cultures are always in transition, they determine, to some extent, the health seeking behaviour of a community. It is therefore important to know the cultural beliefs and practices regarding pregnancy and childbirth within that society to understand why women in a particular society choose a particular care. There are many anthropological and sociological studies that explore these areas.

In many cultures pregnancy and childbirth is seen as a valued but normal physiological state which does not require special care. Although pregnancy, childbirth and immediate post-partum period are considered as the most vulnerable period for both the mother and the baby, it is also a regularly expected event of normal womanhood. Therefore, the event differs from illnesses and many studies show that pregnancy and childbirth are considered as conditions not requiring medical care unless problems arise (Kazmi, 1995; PMMN, 1992; Auerbach, 1982). On the other hand, others perceive it as an extra-ordinary event evolving from spiritual matter (Mutambirwa, 1985; Oosterbaan and Barreto da Costa, 1995).

In rural Nepal, ability to have a child (especially son) is considered as the road for women's security (Acharya, 1997). On the other hand, childbirth is considered as a polluted event (Schutzke, 1998). Mothers-in-law are preferred for delivery care rather than trained TBA who were considered expensive (Steinmann and Ramji, 1996).

2.4.3.2 Community risk perceptions and perceptions of illness aetiology regarding pregnancy and childbirth

The objective of the risk approach in antenatal care is to identify women at risk and provide special care to those in need (WHO, 1978). To accomplish this objective the service must be able to pick up women at risk and the women who received advice should follow the advice given. Moreover, appropriate care must be given to those who were identified. However, this is not the case as seen in many studies. Many authors realise the importance of community's perception on risk, severity and causation of illness (Jahn and Kowalewski 1998; Dujardin et al. 1995; Thaddeus and Maine, 1994) and call to re-assess and re-pack the risk package (Villar and Bergsjo, 1997; McDonagh, 1996; Rooney, 1992).

In the context of complications related to pregnancy and childbirth, Thaddeus and Maine (1994) point out that the prospective health care users must recognise the abnormal condition in order to seek care. This is influenced by the prevalence of the condition, perception of risks, perceived severity and causation of illness. Anthropological studies from Guinea-Bissau and Korea have shown that perception of risk is related to cultural beliefs, modified by knowledge on medically defined risks (Oosterbaan and Barreto da Costa, 1995; Sich, 1988). Childbirth was seen as a matter of competing spirits of mother and child in rural Guinea-Bissau. In some parts of western Africa, small bleeding during pregnancy and prolonged labour (up to 2-3 days) are not considered as a matter of concern (PMMN, 1992).

When abnormal conditions during pregnancy and childbirth are recognised and perceived as severe enough to seek care, the perceived causation of illness becomes an important factor to choose where to seek care. The community perception on causation of illness is influenced by the culture. The idea of impurity invading the body in cases of obstetric complications and a subsequent need to clean was common in Bangladesh (Bhatia, 1981), some western African cultures (Oosterbaan and Barreto da Costa, 1995; PMMN, 1992) and in Zimbabwe (Mutambirwa, 1985). Therefore, care from traditional healers and diviners is sought before consulting modern medical care. However, care sought simultaneously for an illness: somatic care from modern medicine and spiritual care from traditional healers, is common among many communities in transition (Kowalewski et al 1998).

2.4.3.3 Value and status of women in the society

Women's status is the interrelation of educational, cultural, economical, legal and political position of women in a given society. Internationally, emphasis has been put on increasing women empowerment and improving their status in a given society. However, in many societies, women are still suffering from the consequences of inequality and inequity due to discriminations, which may even start in their foetal life as in China and India.

The woman's status determines her access to health care, her health care behaviour and her health status, which are the immediate factors that determine the likelihood of death from pregnancy related conditions (McCarthy and Maine, 1992). Moreover, women's autonomy and status within the family as well as the community were found to be related with their ability to decide, and the consequent health service utilisation (Bhatia and Cleland, 1995; Csete, 1993; Okafor, 1991; Nougtara et al. 1989). On the other hand, women are dying outside health service from obstetric complications due to the fact that they were not allowed to go out of their compound in the absence of their husband (PMMN, 1992).

2.4.3.4 Perspectives of community on modern health services

Community or individual perspectives on the health care provided by various providers is a basic factor influencing utilisation of a particular service. The perception of health services is moulded by previous experiences and the perceived quality of care. From the experience from the PMMN in western Africa, Maine (1997) emphasises that community or culture should not be blamed for non-utilisation of health services. It was shown that people do not use services that do not meet their expectation. Similar findings were reported earlier in rural Burkina Faso where mothers chose to walk to the nearest dispensary for ANC to see a midwife instead of seeing village health worker from the same village (Nougtara et al. 1989) and in rural Guatemala where health services were not used due to their inability to fulfil the community's expectation (Annis, 1981). Studies show that hospitals were not used for delivery care even in cases of complications because they were not perceived as a safe place (Kazmi, 1995; Oosterbaan and Barreto da Costa, 1995; Dehne et al. 1995).

2.5 Summary of literature on assessing the safe motherhood programmes

Experiences have shown that:

- The focus on maternal health in developing countries is a recent event that has been originating from a high discrepancy of maternal mortality between developed and developing countries and the realisation that this tragedy could be prevented.

- The effectiveness of maternity care services in developing countries in preventing maternal death is doubtful and depends on a variety of factors. To be effective, the services must be organised in a way that it is available and accessible. In addition, the service must provide good quality care so that the community accepts the service, makes use of it and thus enables the service to have an impact on the community's health.

- The community perspectives on pregnancy and childbirth as well as on modern health service play an important role in the utilisation of maternity care services.

- For rural Nepal exists little knowledge in the area of "quality of maternity care services".

3 Material and Methods

3.1 Introduction

This chapter presents the methodology used in the study. The study area, study design, the main characteristics of the study population, the data collection procedure including the general procedures, instruments for data collection and sources of data, the data recording and the data analysis procedures, feedback to the community and lastly the main limitations and sources of bias are presented.

3.2 Short description of the study area

The study was done in the Banke district, situated in the *terai* part (plain) of mid-western development region and near the Indian border (*see annex 1a & 1b*). The total population of Banke district for the year 1996/97 is estimated to be approximately 338,000 (projection from 1991 census) with an urban population of 56,600 and a rural population of 281,400. Expected deliveries in the district were 13,520, with the estimated crude birth rate of 40/1000 population. The district covers one municipality and 46 village development committees (VDC). One VDC covers 9 wards which are composed of a number of villages depending on the size of population in the villages.

Nepalganj is the district municipal town of Banke district. There is one government hospital, one private hospital, 2 government primary health centres, 10 government health posts and 30 government sub-health posts in the district. According to the latest national family health survey, the crude coverage of ANC in this mid-western *Terai* was 29.1% and professionally assisted delivery was 7.7%.

3.3 Study design

3.3.1 Study methods and data sources

The study comprises two parts: a cross sectional study of selected health facilities and a community based qualitative study.

The quantitative assessment of antenatal and obstetric care services was done following the three steps as defined by Donabedian namely structural, process and output quality. Availability and accessibility of services are assessed as the structural quality, performance of health services and actual utilisation as the process quality, institution-based mortality rates and user satisfaction as the output quality. Additional assessment was done on communities' perspectives regarding care in pregnancy and delivery to enrich factors determining use of maternal health care services.

Quantitative methods were applied to find out the actual situation of health services infrastructure, actual use of antenatal and obstetric care services and performance of health service on antenatal and obstetric care. A predetermined set of indicators was used as a tool to assess the quality. Both quantitative and qualitative approaches were applied to determine factors determining use of maternal health care services and communities' perception on modern health care services related to antenatal and obstetric care.

Descriptive studies collect information about people (service) which are analysed in categories of attributes and variables. They are mainly observational and are carried out as cross-sectional or longitudinal studies (Kirkwood, 1988, p. 153-160).

The following data sources were used.
1. Review of documents.
2. Inventories of building, equipment, drugs, supplies and staff in public health services, with respect to the stated objectives.
3. Observation of health worker's performance by observation of 58 antenatal consultations in 13 units.
4. Interviews with health workers (n=19).
5. Exit interviews with antenatal care attendees (n = 136).
6. Interview with hospital maternity patients (n = 146).
7. Focus group discussions with women, 6 focus group with 56 participants.
8. Key-informant interviews (n = 21).

Details of data collection procedures will be presented in 3.3.

3.3.2 Study targets and selection of health facilities

The study frame includes all modern health facilities with maternal health care services in Banke district, documents and registers from last year (1996/97), the service providers, the service users and the communities. However, women and health services beyond Rapti river were not included due to inaccessibility during the study period.

Material and methods

The government and private hospitals in Nepalganj were included. The health post at the hospital compound was chosen purposively because it is the only FLHS that provides antenatal care for the urban population. A random sample of 13 rural health centres with maternal health care services were selected.

A stratified random sampling method was applied. The health centres were stratified according to their level, PHC and HP in one group and SHP in another group. The health centres not providing antenatal care service and those beyond the Rapti river were not included in the sampling frame. A random sample was selected from each sampling frame (see below) with the help of table of random number, Fisher and Yates, 1963 (Kirkwood, 1988, p. 221-224). The sample comprised one PHC, 3 HP and 9 SHP (see below). The nearest one was 3 Km and the furthermost one was 60 Km from Nepalganj. Most facilities lay 1-6 Km distance from the major road except Holiya, Belahari and Kamdi. The catchment population of the sampled facilities is 154000 with 6160 expected deliveries in 1996/97. The sampling frame and selected facilities are presented in table 1 (see P. 32)

3.4 Data collection

Data collection was done from 06.06.97 to 12.09.97 by the researcher with the help of interviewers. Document analysis, observation of health workers' performance and interviews with health workers and key-informants were done by the researcher herself with the help of a translator. A translator was required for observation of the conversation between health workers and the clients. Antenatal exit interviews were done by three interviewers. The hospital maternity interviews were done by one separate interviewer. The focus group discussions were facilitated by the principle interviewer and note taking was done by another interviewer. They were specially trained for this purpose.

Interviewees were informed about the purpose of the study and asked for a verbal agreement to the interview itself and the tape-recording procedure for focus group discussion. The interviews were performed in a special room or under a tree and confidentiality was assured to each interviewee. Privacy was assured whenever possible. Many facilities were visited two or three times as the low utilisation of the service made it difficult to achieve the required number of interviewees.

Demographic data of the district was obtained from the district public health office (DPHO) and the district development committee (DDC) office, Information and Sociology department, Banke district. Information on distance of villages covered by the health facility with their population were obtained from health workers or village development committee members of respective FLHS.

Table 1: Sampling frame with selected facilities* and their catchment population

First line health services	Catchment population	First line health services	Catchment population
1. Bankatwa PHC	14054	6. Hirminiya SHP	6237
2. Bagheswari HP	11530	**7. Holiya SHP**	**5396**
3. Jaishpur HP	4989	8. Inderapur SHP	6396
4. Kanchanapur HP	**6475**	**9. Kamdi SHP**	**7156**
5. Samsherganj HP	**5777**	10. Khaskusma SHP	4545
6. Sonpur HP	6571	11. Kohalpur SHP	13128
7. Nepalganj HP**	**56608**	12. Mahadevpuri SHP	8180
Sub-health post		**13. Manikapur SHP**	**6878**
1. Bankatti SHP	4509	**14. Naubasta SHP**	**13211**
2. Belahari SHP	**4157**	**15. Paraspur SHP**	**3789**
3. Belbhar SHP	**4242**	16. Radhapur SHP	6189
4. Betahani SHP	**6150**	17. Sitapur SHP	5167
5. Chisapani SHP	3388	18. Udarapur SHP	7514

* = selected facilities in bold.
** = not included in sampling frame, selected purposively.

3.4.1 Selection and training of interviewers

Selection criteria for interviewers was set as follows,
-female from the area with ability to read and write,
-ability to speak English, *Nepali* and Hindi or a local language,
-willingness to participate in research, and
-not belonging to the health sector.

Material and methods

However, in practice it was difficult to find women able to speak English and the local languages from the area. The principle interviewer was a master student of Sociology from Kathmandu, with experience in doing similar types of research. Two are professional teachers, and another one is an auxiliary nurse midwife but working as laboratory technician at the hospital STD department. All the interviewers except the one who performed maternity interviews speak *Nepali*, Hindi and English and are not from health sector. Two interviewers had experience of doing individual interviews and focus group discussion.

The objectives of the study, the guidelines and the main principles of interview were discussed with them in advance. The main component of training was learning by doing.

3.4.2 Pilot testing

A pilot testing was done during a period of two weeks in two health units, a rural and an urban one. The questionnaires and interview guideline were modified after pilot test concerning understandability, sequence and phrasing. The guideline for key-informant's interviews became more structured, and family planning advice given 'after delivery' was dropped out as the labour room in-charge came to know the contents of questionnaire. The observation guideline was amended.

3.4.3 Data collection instruments

All the data collection tools were developed in Heidelberg with the working group on Health System Research, Reproductive Health, Institute for Tropical Hygiene and Public Health, University of Heidelberg. A set of indicators was developed (*see annex 10*). All the tools were also presented to experts in Kathmandu and Nepalganj and their advice was taken into account when revising the tools. The national maternity care guideline and Standards/Guidelines for Primary Level Health Institutions were used as references.

All instruments for data collection except checklists and key-informant interview guideline were translated into *Nepali* by one translator in Kathmandu and one interviewer. Counterchecks were done with another translator.

Records reviews, inventories of equipment, drugs, supplies and staff, and observations were performed with a pre-formed checklist. Health worker interviews, antenatal exit interviews and maternity interviews were done with structured questionnaires. A semi-structured interview guideline was applied for key-informant interviews with health personnel, community leaders and TBA. Focus group discussions were done with a guideline for discussion containing 5 main topics.

3.4.4 Quantitative data collection

This study is an observational cross-sectional study. Review of documents, inventories of equipment, drugs, supplies and staff, interviews with health service users and providers, and structured observations of health workers' performance were used as quantitative tools.

3.4.4.1 Document reviews

Monthly and annual reports of 2053/54 (1996/97) were reviewed from the district medical officer and district public health offices. The report of the regional review meeting (1996/97) covers 2809 antenatal attendees and 2883 deliveries attended by trained personnel including trained TBA. A pre-formed checklist was applied to review antenatal, delivery and operation registers (*see annex 2a & b*).

The antenatal register was reviewed with a checklist at each FLHS visited whenever available. Data on antenatal attendees (n=1378) was obtained from nine registers which were available for the last year. Others (5 units) said they lost or did not register or did not offer services last year. However, according to other informants, these services started their antenatal care services very recently. 274 antenatal cards from four units who keep antenatal card in the health unit and 136 cards from antenatal attendees were available for review. There was incomplete registration both in antenatal cards and registers.

Antenatal registers from FLHS were reviewed on the following aspects:
- total number of attendees,
- number of first, second and 3+ visits,
- duration of pregnancy at the time of first visit in weeks,
- identified risk factors,
- recorded referral advice, and
- personal data such as age, parity, religion, village in distance of the attendees.

Material and methods 35

80-90% complete data was obtained, except duration of pregnancy at the time of first visit. However, identified risk factors and referral advice are taken as documented.

From hospital and private antenatal care services, only the total number of antenatal care attendees was available. Number of first time attendees from the district in these services was estimated from data of randomly selected 40 women interviewed from hospital antenatal care for other purpose.

Data on institutional delivery care (n=1323) was obtained from both government and private hospital. Birth register was not available in any FLHS visited as they hardly provide institutional delivery care service. Government hospital maternity ward registers were reviewed for different periods due to unavailability of some registers. The birth register was reviewed for one year period (1996-1997). The operation register was reviewed for one year period. However, complete data could only be obtained for a 4 month period due to incomplete registration. Estimation was made for one year coverage of CS from the available 4 months' data, institutional delivery rates and hospital CS rate. Maternity admission and discharge registers were analysed for the same 4 month period to countercheck operation register.

The operation register of the private hospital was reviewed for one year period. Estimated data on vaginal delivery at private hospital was obtained from the Sister in-charge of the hospital as the register was lost during moving of the hospital from the old to a new building.

The hospital delivery book was reviewed for:
- total number of delivery,
- mode of delivery,
- outcome of baby including weight and vital status,
- previous history of still birth and abortion, and
- personal data such as age, parity, distance from the hospital of the maternity cases. Complete data was obtained in 85%.

Operation, maternity admission and discharge registers were reviewed for:
- total number of CS,
- outcome of CS including still birth and maternal death,
- indication for CS, and
- their personal data such as age, parity and distance from the hospital.

These documents were a rich source of information and review and analysis of available documents gave a wide range of information. However, incompleteness of documents is a common feature in this district as in other developing countries and their accuracy is difficult to estimate.

3.4.4.2 Inventories of building, equipment, drugs and consumable

Structural availability is used as an indicator to determine structural quality of maternal health care services in comparison to national guideline. Guided observation was performed with checklists that includes building, equipment, drugs, consumable and staff availability. All checklists were in English.

Four separate checklists were used for FLHS and hospital, namely (1) for facility and equipment of FLHS; (2) for drugs and consumable of FLHS, (3) for hospital labour room and (4) for hospital theatre. The private hospital was not included because it was in the process of moving to a new building (*see annex 3a & b*).

Although the same checklists were applied for all FLHS, some elements were included or not included according to their function and locality. For example, local anaesthetic and episiotomy repair sets were checked only in HP/PHC. Intravenous drips were not checked at the urban health centre as it lies in the hospital compound and does not provide obstetric first aid, and at SHP.

Facility and equipment checklists were rated score 2 if present and functioning properly at the time of assessment, score 1 if present but not functioning, and score 0 if absent. Drugs and supplies were scored 1 if they are present at the time of visit. No effort was put to assess the availability of drugs and supplies outside the visiting time.

3.4.4.3 Observation of health worker's performance

There is a strong recommendation to use observation of health worker performance to assess the process quality of care. Non-participant observation of antenatal care process was carried out for assessing health worker's performance on antenatal care. Special interest was given to specific components of antenatal care namely history taking with first visit, physical examinations, laboratory investigations and counselling.

A maximum of 5 consultations was observed in each facility as increasing numbers just revealed repetition of action. A total of 58 first visits was observed from 13 centres. One centre did not have clients on the day of visit. A re-visit could not be made due to transportation problems.

The researcher and the translator were in the consultation room while the health worker consulted the expectant mother. A checklist was used as a tool for observation (*see annex 4*). The researcher observed the examination and another observer observed the conversation between health worker and the client. The findings were discussed and compiled at the end of the day.

Observational data gives information that could not be obtained through interviews (Patton, 1990, p. 202-205).

3.4.4.4 Interviews with health workers

According to WHO recommendation, structured interviews were carried out to find out knowledge regarding risk screening in antenatal care and management of normal and complicated delivery. Semi-structured interviews were carried out to determine health worker's opinion on the use and non-use of modern health service by expectant women.

A total of 15 health workers from FLHS (9 maternal child health workers, 5 auxiliary nurse midwives, one student nurse) were interviewed to determine their knowledge on antenatal and obstetric care with the help of a structured questionnaire (*see annex 5*). For assessment of knowledge and perception on risk factors three normal conditions were included to overcome politeness biases. The interview was only performed with health workers who are responsible for maternal health care. Four out of 15 health workers interviewed refused to answer on care of normal delivery as they do not provide delivery care service.

Another four individual structured interviews were carried at the hospital maternity ward focusing on the delivery care. All health workers' interviews were conducted by the researcher with a translator. Most interviews lasted for 30-45 minutes.

All health workers were rated similarly as their functions on the task in questions were not different. Most of questions concerning complicated deliveries were hypothetical as most of them never came across complicated delivery.

3.4.4.5 Interviews with health service users

Antenatal exit interviews

Structured interviews were held with antenatal care attendees together with a review of their antenatal cards after the end of ANC process. A structured questionnaire with some open questions was used (*see annex 6*). This is aimed to determine the quality of care received by these women during this and their last visits.

A total of 136 exit interviews was carried out, 102 from rural health units and 34 from the urban health unit, for assessing quality of antenatal care service. At first all attendees or systematic sample of ANC attendees that is every second attendee was included according to the number of attendees. However, in some HC it was not possible to select with systematic sampling and convenient sampling was used: after finishing one interview, the interviewer went to collect the next women or the health worker sent the women to the interviewer. Three interviewees were not included because they left before the end of interview. Interviews were conducted in a separate room or under a tree nearby the health centre. Each interview lasted for 30-40 min. Interviews were done with a structured questionnaire in *Nepali* by three interviewers and translated by the interviewer themselves.

Most facilities provide antenatal care on a particular date of the week/month (e.g. Wednesdays and 17/18 date of *Nepali* month) which caused difficulties in visiting these centres. In most cases revisit were done in order to conduct desired number of interviews.

Maternity interviews

Structured interviews with maternity patients from Bheri zonal hospital at their discharge together with review of their record were done for 3 months. A structured questionnaire with some open questions was used (*see annex 7*). This is aimed to determine the quality of obstetric care received, components of antenatal care and referral practice from the client who went for antenatal care.

A total of 146 maternity patients was interviewed in three month periods. Although 60-80 women from the district delivered every month in this hospital, the interviewer was not able to interview all the patients because many women left the hospital just after delivery (leave against medical advice) and most of these patients were missed. They represent about 20-30% of hospital delivery cases. This could be a source of bias as these women might be different from the rest in their health seeking behaviour as well as their opinion. Each interview lasted for 15-20 minutes. The interview was done with a structured questionnaire in *Nepali* by one interviewer and translated by a translator.

Exit interviews of health services users are widely used to assess the service they recently received, thus overcoming recall bias. Although there could be politeness biases where interviews were held in the vicinity of health facilities, it gives detail of the whole process of care.

3.4.5 Qualitative data collection

Qualitative methods give information on "what exists" and "why it exists". A variety of qualitative methods were used to assess a district health system (Maier et al. 1994, p. 3). In this study qualitative methods, namely focus group discussions and key-informant interviews were applied to explore community's perception on modern maternal health care services, their beliefs and practices and their health seeking behaviour regarding pregnancy and child birth.

3.4.5.1 Focus group discussions

Focus group discussion gives a large body of information within a short period and have self-correcting mechanism. It gives insight into the people's beliefs, perception, attitudes and behaviour. The ideal number of participants is 6-10 with the similar age, sex and socio-cultural back ground. The facilitator and the place should be neutral (Maier et al. 1994, p. 36-43; Patton, 1990, p. 317).

These discussions were conducted in order to gain information on health seeking behaviour during pregnancy and child birth and perceptions of the general population regarding modern antenatal and obstetric care services. This was done as the service users are not a good source of information for identifying the reasons impeding people to attend the health services. Moreover, their viewpoint may differ considerably from the attitudes and behaviour of users of modern health services. Emphasis was put on utilisation and non-utilisation of antenatal and delivery care services and high risk pregnancies including STD and complicated deliveries (*see annex 8*).

Six focus group discussions were carried out with a total of 56 participants in three villages. These villages are with FLHS providing antenatal care and were chosen according to their accessibility to the referral level care.

One female facilitator conducted all the discussions and one female note-taker took notes. Tape recording and observation were done by the researcher. Two focus group discussions were not recorded due to technical problems. All groups were organised with the help of the village development committees. Criteria for participants were women with at least one child from the village and nearby villages. Four groups were performed with Hindu women and two groups with Muslim women, as participants of similar social and family back ground were desirable. Their age was between 19-45 years and number of children was 1-6 children. The discussions were held in *Nepali* and Hindi and lasted 1-1:30 hours. Four groups were done at a school building and two at a village development committee office building. Most women came with their children and there were many disturbances from the children as well as from some curious men and women.

As discussions were held in villages, it was not possible to obey the rule of focus group discussion such as participants not knowing each other. However, most of them participated voluntarily and had the same socio-cultural back ground.

3.4.5.2 Key-informant interviews

Key-informants are people who have a special position in the community and are representatives of the opinion and experiences of a whole group. They give valuable and independent information about the whole community or group and are very useful in complementing focus group discussion (Maier et al. 1994). A total of 21 key-informant interviews was done using a semi-structured guideline (*see annex 9*). The aim was to determine factors deterring use of maternal health care services, namely antenatal care, delivery care and referral level care by expectant women. Key-informants include 3 obstetricians and gynaecologists, three person from DPHO, one TBA, two VDC members, and 12 health centre staff. Most of the interviews were performed during informal talks except those with doctors.

Material and methods

3.5 Feedback to the community

Feedback of preliminary results is a mean of increasing validity. The preliminary result was presented to the district medical officer (DMO), obstetricians, personnel from DPHO office, UNICEF (United Nations Children's Fund), UNFPA (United Nations Association for Population Fund), other international non-governmental organisations working in maternal health care programme and some auxiliary nurse midwives (ANM) and the comments from these personnel were noted for discussion.

3.6 Data recording and analysis

Data on facility checklist was analysed manually for structural quality of maternity care services in Banke district. Data from review of registers was entered and analysed by Microsoft Excel programme for coverage of maternity care services. All antenatal exit and maternity interviews data were entered into Epi Info programme and analysed for information on process quality. Data from health worker interview and observations of health worker's performance were analysed manually for process quality. Chi-square test was applied for testing difference of proportions.

Records from focus group discussions were transcribed and translated by the facilitator and note taker. The control of translation was done by transcription and translation of two tape records by another independent translator. Focus group interviews and key-informant interviews were coded according to the guideline and analysed.

The validity of information obtained was cross-checked by obtaining data from different sources, triangulation. Triangulation is a technique using different techniques in one study to combine strengths and to correct deficiencies of a different technique (Patton, 1990). There are different types of triangulation according to Denzin namely (1) data triangulation: use of a variety of data sources (2) investigator triangulation: use of different researcher (3) theory triangulation: the use of multiple perspectives to interpret a single set of data (4) methodological triangulation: the use of multiple methods to study a problem (quoted by Patton, 1990, p. 187).

In this study triangulation was done with 'data triangulation' by using various data sources and 'methodological triangulation' by using different methods.

3.7 Limitations

- The affiliation of the researcher with the health service must have influenced the interviews, especially regarding use and non-use of modern health services.
- Using non-participant observation to determine the quality of health worker's performances is a source of biases as the awareness of being observed can change the performance and attitude (social desirability). This was seen in better identification of risk pregnancies during the observation. However, this bias was controlled by counterchecking with other source of data (e.g. register).
- Although it is difficult to interpret the knowledge of a health worker with a single structured interview, it gives a rough estimate. The use of knowledge as a proxy indicator for their practice on hospital obstetric care is also a source of biases as knowledge and practice differ obviously with ANC.
- Five out of 14 FLHS did not keep proper record. Therefore, the result obtained from register may be biased towards better performing units.
- The sample excluded women and services beyond Rapti river. Moreover, interviews were not performed with users of private practices. This could have given a more complete picture of health services in the district.
- Privacy during the interviewing process was not obtained in all interviews because of lack of room in the health unit together with the limitation of the monsoon season. Moreover, exit interviews performed in the proximity of health facilities could not rule out politeness biases.
- Selection of participants of the focus group discussions was done through village development committees that have a close connection with FLHS and with the management committee. These double connections can influence the findings. Disturbances from children and others may also have influenced the participants especially when discussing on traditional practices and non-use of services.
- Translation biases like in every study done in places foreign to the researcher, is one of the greatest sources of bias. However, a countercheck was done whenever necessary to overcome this problem.
- Furthermore, inability to obtain complete data like in maternity interviews and CS data may have influenced the result.

4 Results

4.1 The state of maternal health care infrastructure in Banke district, Nepal

4.1.1 Availability of antenatal and obstetric care services in the district

The total population of Banke district for the year 1996/97 is estimated to be approximately 338,000 with expected deliveries of 13,520. There is one public hospital in Nepalganj covering for Bheri zone (5 districts, one of which is Banke district) and one private hospital capable of doing Caesarean section. There are 42 first line health facilities in the district including 2 primary health centres (PHC), 10 health posts (HP) and 30 sub-health posts (SHP). The number of staff allocated in PHC is 12, in HP is 8 or 9, and in SHP is 4.

4.1.1.1 Service outlets

ANC service was provided at one urban FLHS, the hospital out-patient department and 3 private clinics in the urban area and at 27 out of 41 (66%) rural FLHS of the district.

Although 35 out of 42 FLHS had female health workers capable of providing maternal health care, ANC was only provided by 28 FLHS at the time of the study. 17 facilities provided static services and 20 facilities provided outreach service at about 100 outreach points[1]. Absence of ANC was mostly due to the lack of female health workers. Another reason mentioned was that 'women do not come for ANC here, they go to town', by one HP with no maternal health care service.

The availability of FLHS was 1 facility per 8000 population. However, FLHS offering ANC was 1 facility per 12000 inhabitants.

ANC was also provided by medical doctors at the hospital out-patient department 5 days per week, 3-4 hours a day, functioning as a first line health service. There was no referral system functioning in the district. Every women can have access to doctors' ANC (out-patient department) without any referral from FLHS. There was no discrimination between referred and non-referred cases (in terms of waiting time or fees). There are 3 private clinics (providing

---

[1] Antenatal care was provided by MCHW at 5 different villages of the catchment area.

ANC) run by medical doctors. Their opening time varies from 5-7 hours per day, 6 days per week.

Delivery care was mainly provided by family members and relatives. TBA and staff from 16 FLHS also provided home delivery services. Institutional deliveries were mainly confined to two hospitals in Nepalganj.

Two hospitals in Nepalganj are providing essential obstetric care as defined by WHO (1991a). Caesarean section can be done at both government and private hospitals on a 24 hours basis.

4.1.1.2 Health manpower

Availability of staff in the district was obtained from the district public health nurse and hospital nurses in-charge.

Professional health workers

There are 26 medical doctors (government 18 & private 8) practising in the district and 6 surgeons are capable of doing CS.

There are 16 trained staff (staff nurse & auxiliary nurse midwife) in government service for providing maternal health care. 10 are posted in HP and PHC and are responsible for providing maternal health care services including both antenatal and obstetric care. The other 6 are stationed at the maternity ward of the Bheri zonal hospital and do not provide ANC. Although trained staff were posted in all health posts and primary health centres, no trained staff worked in the areas beyond Rapti river, at the time of assessment.

There are 27 MCHW (maternal child health workers) in the district. They were trained over a 3-month period, posted in SHP and responsible for both antenatal and basic obstetric care services.

Out of 42 FLHS in the district 7 units did not have trained female health workers (ANM/MCHW) at the time of assessment. Some centres were not allocated yet and some staff were working in other areas.

Trained traditional birth attendants

TBA are included as a health man power due to their role in maternal health care delivery in Nepal. According to DPHO there are 291 traditional birth attendants who got 10 days training in basic maternal health care. However, according to report from FLHS there are 265 trained TBA practising in the district in basic maternal health care. There are also traditional healers practising in the district, however assessment of traditional healers' services was not included in this study.

The following table shows availability of different level of health care personnel per population in the district.

Table 2: Availability of health manpower, Banke district

Availability of health man power	Number of health personnel	Population per health personnel	Expected deliveries/year per health personnel
Trained TBA	265	1275	51
Trained staff (MCHW/ ANM/ staff nurse)	43	7860	314
Trained midwife (ANM/staff nurse)	16	21125	845
Surgeon capable of CS	6	56333	2253

4.1.2 Availability of antenatal and obstetric care services in the selected facilities

4.1.2.1 Health service outlets

At the time of assessment, out of 14 selected FLHS, 6 provided ANC at the station and the outreach points, 6 at the centre and 2 at the outreach points. Consultation for ANC was provided 1-4 days per month (mean 2/month) with opening hours of 3-7 hours per day (mean 3.8 hours).

Not all FLHS providing ANC do provide delivery care. According to national guidelines, HP and PHC have the capability of providing delivery care at health centres. Only two centres (one HP and one PHC) said they provide delivery care at the facility. Home delivery was offered by 11 out of 14 staff interviewed (78.6%). However only 7 staff went for home delivery at night time. All MCHW (SHP staff) interviewed provided home delivery care service. 121

trained TBA provided care during pregnancy and home delivery in the catchment area of selected FLHS.

4.1.2.2 Health manpower

There are 16 female staff including 2 staff nurses, 5 ANM and 9 MCHW who are responsible for maternal health care in 14 FLHS visited.

4.1.2.3 Availability of essential equipment, drugs and consumable in the selected 14 FLHS

Availability of equipment, drugs and consumable was assessed at 14 facilities with the help of a checklist. Emphasis was made on essential basic equipment necessary for antenatal and delivery care such as room with privacy, fetoscope, antenatal card, tape measure, chloroquine, ferrous tablet, iv line and ergometrine injection (see annex 3a). In general, almost all FLHS are to some extent equipped for ANC and more than half of them with drugs and supplies and for providing home delivery care.

On average, 66% of drugs, vaccines and consumable were available at the time of assessment, 62% in SHP and 72% in HP. For essential equipment 67% of 11 items assessed for ANC (in SHP 63% and in HP 75%) and 52% of items assessed for delivery care (14 items for HP/PHC, 9 items for SHP) were present and well functioning at the time of assessment. Screening test for anaemia, urine albumin, urine sugar and for syphilis were not available in all HP/PHC (SHP do not provide according to national guideline).

Table 3 (p. 47) presents availability of individual drug, vaccine and consumable for antenatal and delivery care in all FLHS. Table 4 (p. 48) presents individual achievement of selected FLHS on drugs and supplies and on equipment for antenatal and delivery care. Less than 60% is categorised as poor, 61-80% as accepted, and more than 81% as good.

4.1.2.4 Availability of equipment, drugs and consumable in the referral hospital

Different checklists were used to assess availability of essential equipment, drugs and consumable in government hospital labour room and theatre. In both checklists, emphasis was put on essential equipment, drugs and consumable necessary for complicated delivery care and new born resuscitation such as: vacuum and forceps extractor, adult and new born ambulatory bag, syntocinon injection, intravenous line, oxygen, and morphine. (see annex 3b) Availability of essential equipment, drugs and consumable in government hospital labour room and theatre is presented below (see table 5, p. 48).

Table 3: **Availability of essential drugs, vaccine and consumable at selected 14 FLHS**

SN	Items	Number of FLHS expected to have following items*	% of FLHS with available essential drugs and supplies
1	Contraceptive pills	14	100
2	Tetanus toxiod	14	100
3	Sterile syringes & needles	14	100
4	Intravenous fluid for replacement	4	100
5	Intravenous set	4	100
6	Paracetamol or Aspirin	14	92
7	Chloroquine (oral)	14	79
8	Local anaesthetics (injection)	5	60
9	Antihypertensive drugs (oral)	5	60
10	Iron tablets	14	57
11	Folic acid (oral)	14	36
12	Ergometrine (injection)	14	29
13	Silver nitrate (antibiotics) eye drops	14	29
14	Sterile gloves	14	21

* = *number varies according to their function and locality (urban FLHS is in the hospital compound and does not provide obstetric first aid)*

Table 4: Individual achievement of selected FLHS on drugs and supplies and on equipment for antenatal and delivery care

% of expected achievement	Facilities with % of available drugs and supplies	Facilities with % of available equipment (antenatal care)	Facilities with % of available equipment (delivery care)
< 60%	4	3	9
61-80%	7	8	5
> 81%	3	3	0

Table 5: Availability of essential equipment, drugs and consumable at labour room and theatre, government hospital

Items at:	Scores achieved	% achieved
Labour room (scores n = 22)	15	68%
Theatre (scores n = 22)	18	82%
Total (scores = 44)	33	75%

4.1.3 Accessibility of antenatal and obstetric care services
4.1.3.1 Geographical accessibility

Geographical accessibility of selected 14 first line health services

Each facility has a defined catchment area and population. Most FLHS are easily accessible for the population in most parts of the district. Based on 1991 census data and village covered, almost 90% of population are within 5 Km radius from the facility (see table 6, p. 49). However, facilities providing ANC have to cover more than their catchment population due to facilities not offering ANC services. This means accessibility to antenatal services is more difficult than accessibility of FLHS.

Out of 136 antenatal clients interviewed, most of them came to the facility by walking (73%) or by bicycle (11%) as there is no public transport connecting villages in most areas. Travelling time ranges from 2 minutes to 4 hours. 92% of women walked for less than 1 hour to reach the facility. Others (8%) walked for more than 1 hour to reach the facility. Table 7 shows distance covered by users to reach antenatal care service with their means of transport.

Average cost of transport was 7 *Nepali* Rupees[2] (range = 2-15 Rupees) among 23 women who paid for transport. The minimum daily wages for a labourer is 90 Rupees.

Table 6: Geographical accessibility of selected 14 FLHS

Distance from FLHS	Expected deliveries	%
<= 5 Km	5516	89.5
6-10 Km	531	8.6
> 10 Km	113	1.8
Total	6160	100.0

Table 7: Distance vs. means of transport used by antenatal attendees (n = 135)

Distance	Walking	Rickshaw*	Bicycle	Tempo**	Bus
<= 5 Km	93	17	13	2	0
> 5 Km	5	0	2	2	1
total in %	73%	13%	11%	3%	<1%

*tri-cycle (public transport)
**three-wheel car (public transport)

Geographical accessibility of the referral level obstetric care

The district is situated in the plain region of the country. However, accessibility to the referral level hospital is rather difficult as the district covers a wide area (2337 sq. Km) and public transport is available only for some villages. The furthest FLHS is 80 Km from the hospital. Travel time ranges from 15 minutes to 1-2 days depending on the availability of transport and the season. According to information from the DDC and DPHO office, 45% of population live within

---

[2] *Nepali* Rupees (1 US$ = 56 Nepali Rupees)

10 Km distance from the hospital, 43% between 11-30 Km distance and 12% more than 30 Km distance (see table 8).

The region beyond the Rapti river with 16% of the district population is cut off from the hospital during Monsoon which lasts at least 3 months a year. However, because there is no border control between Nepal and India people from these areas can travel to get emergency medical care at a nearby town in India.

Table 8: Accessibility of referral level hospital, Banke district

Distance from hospital	Population	Expected deliveries	%
<= 10 Km	153120	6125	45
11-30 Km	145135	5805	43
> 30 Km	39745	1590	12
Total	338000	13520	100

source: DDC, Banke district, Nepalganj (projection from 1991 census)

4.1.3.2 Financial accessibility

Financial accessibility of antenatal care services

Most of ANC services are free of charge. Out of 136 attendees interviewed, 62% got free consultation. The other 38% contribute 1-5 Rupees (mean 6.7 for three visits). ANC in hospital out-patient department is more expensive because every woman undergoes laboratory investigation (test for syphilis, Haemoglobin estimation, blood grouping and urine test) with fees amounting up to 100 Rupees in one visit, including the test. TT injection is free and iron tablets is not covered by the service fees.

The amount of money they spent for drugs (e.g. ferrous sulphate) varies greatly depending on the availability of the drugs. The money spent for iron tablets ranges from 4-170 Rupees (mean 88) for one month iron tablets, depending on whether they bought the drug at a health centre or a local market, in comparison to the minimum daily wages of 90 Rupees per day for unskilled labourers (according to DDC). In those cases where the health workers opened a drug store in the same village iron tablets were not given at the HC, in spite of drugs being available at the facility.

Results

Financial accessibility of hospital delivery care services

Delivery care in the government hospital is rather expensive. Although the price of vaginal delivery at the hospital was fixed at 120 Rupees, the total cost incurred by maternity patients interviewed for vaginal delivery care (n = 126) ranged from 300-3000 Rupees (mean 640) including drugs, material and other expenses such as food.

Cost of CS was fixed at 720 Rupees. Total cost spent for CS (n = 20) ranges from 1000-13000 Rupees (mean 5360) including service fees, purchasing materials and drugs and other expense such as food. The cost of transport (n = 137) spent ranges from 4-600 Rupees (mean 35) depending on distance and availability of transport. Cost of transport was higher for women who used ambulance and came from a distance more than 10 Km. The cost presented above do not include opportunity costs for the clients and their families.

The money generated from hospital and out-patient services is used for salary of locally recruited staff (one in three staff at the hospital are locally recruited staff) and for purchasing necessary materials and equipment for the hospital.

4.1.3.3 Socio-cultural accessibility

No major cultural barrier could be identified from the health service side. Most of the health workers as well as doctors providing maternal health care services are women which is appropriate for the culture and also almost all FLHS health workers come from the area and speak the local language. Traditional beliefs and practices regarding pregnancy and delivery are presented in section 4.3 in more detail.

4.2 The state of maternal health care delivery in Banke district

The state of maternal health care delivery will be presented as (1) the actual coverage of maternal health care, (2) the quality of health service performances, (3) the outcome of maternal health care at referral level, (4) co-ordination and supervision among health workers, (5) In-service training of health workers, and (6) community involvement in health care delivery.

4.2.1 Coverage of maternal health care
4.2.1.1 Antenatal care

Based on the first antenatal attendance data from FLHS, hospital and private doctors, ANC coverage was estimated as 28.0% for the whole district. This is almost identical with the finding from Nepal family health survey (NFHS), 1996 i.e. 29.1%. There was a big difference between coverage for urban and rural population, 49.5% and 23.7% respectively.

Antenatal coverage by first line health services and by distance

Antenatal registers reviewed from selected FLHS covered 1378 first antenatal consultations in the year 1996/97, from 9 facilities. Most of antenatal attendees (87%) came from within 5 Km distance from the service and coverage within 5 Km distance was approximately 22%. However, it was not possible to assess exact coverage by distance because of unavailability of catchment population due to absence of ANC services in many FLHS. Table 9, p. 53 (presents the coverage of ANC by individual FLHS (n = 9). There is wide difference from 12.1% to 75.2%. It is interesting to note that the utilisation of ANC services is not affected by the level of health care services.

Coverage by age and parity

Most attendees were from the younger age group which was also found in other studies. The same principle was found for order of pregnancies. Women with less previous pregnancies were more likely to attend ANC than women with more previous pregnancies (see table 10 & 11, p. 53 & 54).

Coverage by religion

ANC Coverage for women from different religions (n = 642) revealed that there was no significant difference between Hindu and Muslim women. It was 27.9% for Hindu and 26.9% for Muslim.

Intensity of use

Most women attended ANC only once and the average number of visits was 1.4 per pregnancy. Only 6% of pregnant women attended ANC for 3 or more times. The valid coverage of ANC (3+ visit in one pregnancy) was only 1.7%.

Results

Timeliness of care

This data derived from 274 antenatal cards reviewed from 4 facilities and 131 antenatal cards reviewed from exit interviews (total = 405). Most first antenatal consultation took place after 20 weeks of gestation, 37.5% before 20 weeks of gestation and 9.4% after 36 weeks of gestation (see table 12, p. 54).

Table 9: Coverage of antenatal care by individual FLHS

Name of FLHS	Coverage of antenatal care
Paraspur SHP	75.2%
Kohalpur SHP	40.8%
Nepalganj HP	29.6%
Sonpur HP	28.5%
Betahani SHP	27.2%
Samsherganj HP	25.5%
Kanchanapur HP	24.7%
Kamdi SHP	14.9%
Bankatwa PHC	12.1%
Sub-total all SHP	**36.0%**
Sub-total all HP & PHC	**26.2%**

Table 10: Antenatal coverage by age of women in selected 14 FLHS (n = 1378)

Age at antenatal visit	% of age group among antenatal visit	% of age group among expected deliveries*	Antenatal coverage of age group
<= 19 year	25.7	18.7	30.5%
20 - 34	69.8	71.6	21.6%
>=35	4.4	9.7	10.1%
Total	100%	100%	22.2%

* source = Pradhan et al. (1996)

Table 11: Antenatal coverage by number of gestation in selected 14 FLHS (n = 1371)

Number of gestation at visit	% among antenatal attendees	% among population*	Coverage by gestation
G 1	43.5	23.0	42.0
G 2-3	41.6	38.5	24.0
G >= 4	15.0	38.5	8.7

* source = Pradhan et al. (1996)
Pregnancy >= 4 was used as high risk pregnancy by national guideline. According to international cut off point gravid (G) >= 6, coverage of multi-parity was 5.1%.

Table 12: Weeks of gestation at 1st antenatal visit from AN card review (n = 405)

Weeks of gestation at 1st visit	Number of first attendees	% of first attendees
<= 20 weeks	152	37.5
21-35 weeks	215	53.1
>= 36 weeks	38	9.4

4.2.1.2 Delivery care

Hospital registers review covered 1323 deliveries in the year 1996/97. This means 9.8% of expected deliveries from the district took place at the hospitals. 1168 women delivered vaginally and 155 by CS. Hospital CS rate was 11.7% and population based CS rate was 1.1%.

Delivery care was also provided at two FLHS in the district but was not registered. FLHS staff assisted an average of 3 (1-5) home deliveries per months. Based on this data they cover about 6% of total expected deliveries in the district which is in line with 5.4% for the area of NFHS data, 1996. Another 18% of expected deliveries in the district were assisted by trained TBA at home. Reported number of deliveries assisted by trained TBA varied greatly. Other deliveries were taking place at home without medically trained assistance (see table 13, p. 55).

Results

Obstetric coverage by place of origin

Out of 13520 expected deliveries from the district 1323 deliveries took place at the hospitals in the year 1996/97. Coverage of hospital delivery for urban area was 36% and for rural area was 4.5%. The hospital delivery rate as well as CS rate for women coming from more than 10 Km distance was 10 times less than from within 10 Km distance (see table 14).

Obstetric coverage by age and parity

Out of hospital deliveries, most women were nulliparous (44.1%) and age group of between 20-30 years (69%). Multi-parity (G 6+) represent only 2.2% with the coverage of 1.4% for the whole district (table 15 & 16, p. 56).

Table 13: Coverage of delivery by health care providers, Banke district

Provider of health care	Coverage of delivery by provider of care (%)	Coverage of delivery by provider of care (%)
Trained TBA (home)	18.0	55.7**
FLHS staff (home)	6.0	5.4*
Hospitals	9.8	4.3*
Home deliveries without medically trained assistant	66.2***	34.6*

*= Pradhan et al. (1996), data for mid-western *Terai*
**= medically trained & un-trained TBA
***= calculation from above data

Table 14: Coverage of hospital delivery and population based CS rate by distance, Banke district

Distance from hospital	coverage of hospital deliveries (n = 1323) (%)	Pop. based C-section rate (n = 155) (%)
<= 10 Km	19.3	2.3
> 10 Km	1.9	0.2
Total (district)	9.8	1.1

Table 15: Coverage of hospital delivery by age (n = 1320)

Age of women at birth	% of age group among hospital deliveries	% of age group among expected deliveries*	Coverage %
<= 19 year	18.6	18.7	9.8
20-34 year	74.5	71.6	10.2
>= 35 year	6.8	9.7	6.9
Total	100	100%	9.8

* Source = Pradhan et al. (1996)

Table 16: Coverage of hospital delivery by number of gestations (n = 1320)

Number of gestations	% among hospital deliveries	% among expected deliveries*	Coverage %
G 1	44.2	23.0	18.8
G 2-3	42.0	38.5	10.7
G 4+	13.8	38.5	3.5

* Source = Pradhan et al. (1996)

4.2.1.3 Post-natal care

There was no record to check the practice of post-natal care. During visits to FLHS, no woman who came for post-natal check up was encountered. However, from interviews, health workers re-visited after 24 hours of home delivery.

4.2.2 Health service performances

This data derived from observation of 58 antenatal consultations at different facilities, structured interviews with 19 health workers, 136 antenatal exit interviews, 146 maternity patient interviews, review of antenatal registers and hospital registers.

Results

4.2.2.1 Knowledge of health workers excluding TBA

A short knowledge test was done with 15 FLHS staff and 4 hospital staff on components of ANC especially on risk screening, and care of normal delivery, new born and complicated deliveries namely post-partum haemorrhage and prolonged labour.

Average knowledge of FLHS staff was presented below (see figure 1, below). Knowledge of hospital staff on components of delivery care including care of new born was 83% of expected knowledge. The most frequent contents health workers failed to mention in care of normal delivery were reviewing antenatal cards (100%) and monitoring of post-partal blood loss (72%). In regards to care of prolonged labour, giving antibiotics (100%), emptying bladder (93%) and assessing vital signs (60%) were not well covered. Emptying bladder (93%), massage of uterus or bi-manual compression (93%) and assessing vital signs (67%) were not well known in case of post-partum haemorrhage (PPH).

Figure 1: Knowledge of FLHS staff on antenatal and obstetric care (n=15)

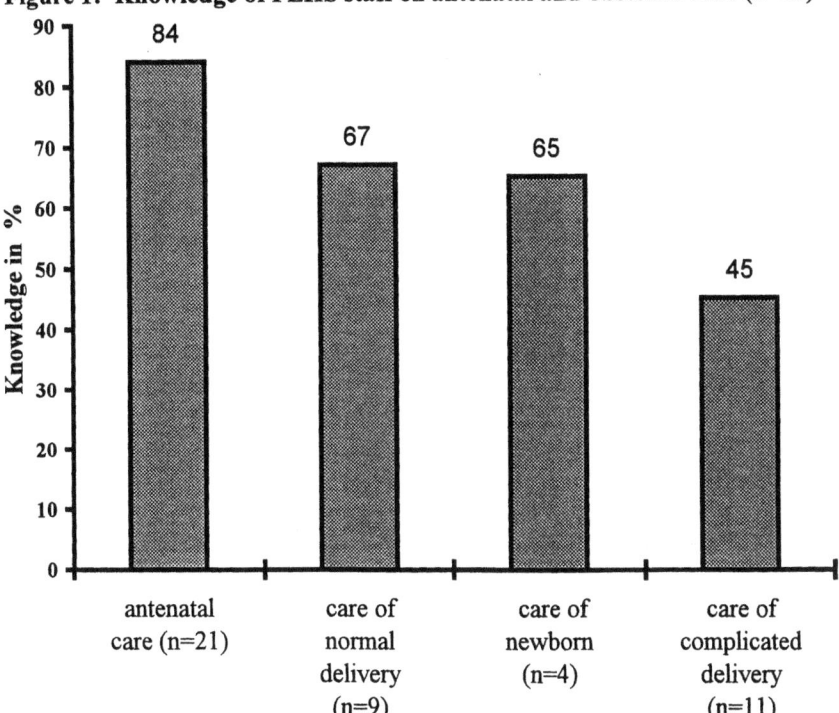

4.2.2.2 Performance of health workers on preventive and promotive activities of ANC

Consultation and counselling time

Among 58 consultations observed, the average duration of consultation was 10 minutes (5-15 minutes). Most of the consultation time was for history taking, examination and form filling. Average individual counselling time was less than one minute ranging from no counselling to four minutes period counselling.

Health education and counselling

57% of 14 FLHS staff interviewed hold group health education sessions for pregnant women. Most of them were taking place in outreach programmes. One group health education was organised in one centre during the visits.

Out of 58 consultations observed, the most frequent contents of counselling and advice were assurance to the women, personal hygiene and nutrition. The communication was mainly one-way, with patients listening to what the health workers said. The women's social situation was never inquired (see figure 2).

Figure 2: Proportion of antenatal attendees advised/counselled (n = 58)

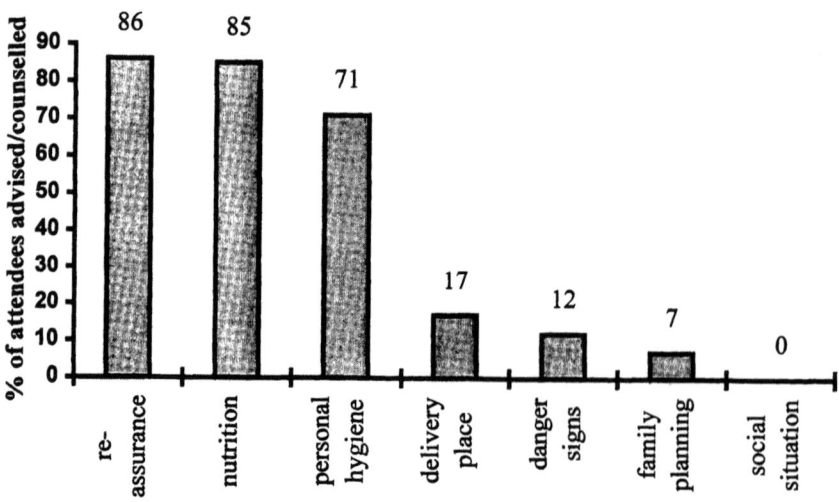

More or less similar picture was observed in antenatal exit interview. About 69% of women interviewed (n = 136) reported to have received at least one health advice in the course of their antenatal consultation concerning aspects of nutrition, iron tablet dose, danger signs and family planning (see table 17). Out of 136 antenatal interviewees, 29% got time to ask question, 65% had no time to ask questions and the rest did not have any question to ask. 56% of women were asked to come back for another check-up.

Table 17: Contents of health education given to antenatal attendees (n=136)

Contents of health education	Number of women who got information	%
Nutrition (n = 136)	88	65
Iron tablet dosage (n = 59)	31	53
Danger sign (n = 136)	20	15
Family planning (n = 134)	12	9

Effectiveness of health education and counselling

As it was difficult to assess effectiveness of these activities, knowledge of antenatal attendees was used as a proxy for effectiveness of these activities. Health education was rated as effective if interviewee able to reproduce contents of health education (danger signs) told during this antenatal visit. 60% of women, who reported to have received information on danger signs were able to reproduce at least one danger sign. 48% of ANC attendees did not know the recommended minimum number of ANC visits in one pregnancy and 28% answer 3 or more visits. 17% of women knew the benefit of tetanus vaccination correctly. Others attributed the following benefits: preventing polio, preventing curved leg of baby, and better health of both mother and baby.

Anaemia prophylactics

32% of antenatal attendees interviewed (n = 136) received a prescription of iron tablets with this visit. Out of 20 women who received prescription with previous visit, only 65% received the drugs and all said to take all the drugs they received irrespective of duration. 5 (25%) women got the drugs free of charge from the service, 8 (40%) women bought from the services as well as from local market. 7 women did not buy the drugs because they were not explained the benefit of the drugs (n = 2) or lack of money (n = 5).

Among hospital deliveries interviewed (n = 146), 25% received iron tablets during their ANC and 90% of them took iron tablets more than 30 days during this pregnancy. 30 days was used as minimum days of Iron tablets needed for effective results. The average duration of oral iron supplement was 53 days (15-150 days).

Based on the data of 28% antenatal coverage, 32% prescription rate and 65% who actually received drugs from antenatal exit interviews and 90% who took >= 30 days iron tablets in this pregnancy among maternity interviews, the following graph can be derived regarding population based coverage of anaemia prophylactics in pregnancy.

Figure 3: Population based coverage of anaemia prophylactics in pregnancy

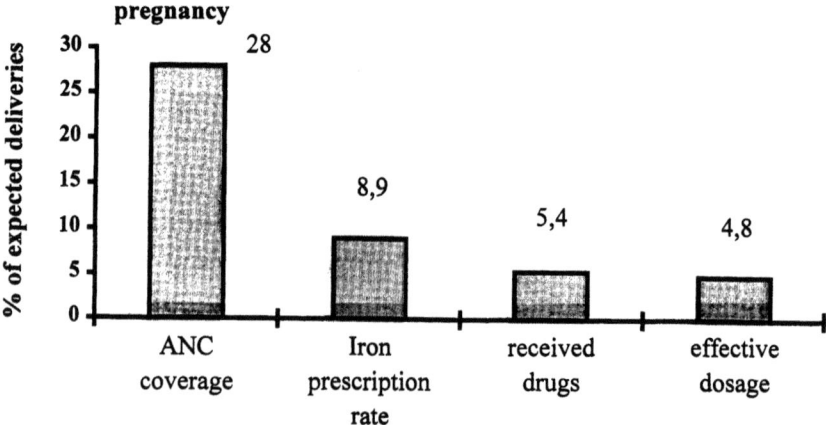

Looking at the given graph, the most pitfall area lies within the health service. The women comply fairly well with medication as long as they received the medicine and got explanations about the benefits of medicine and dosage.

Tetanus prophylactics

In Nepal, 5 doses of Tetanus Toxoid injection (TT) was recommended to all women of reproductive age (15-44 years) for live long protection. Crude coverage for two doses of TT was 12.4% and 5 doses was <5% for the district. However, coverage of two doses of TT among antenatal attendees (n = 136) was 51.4% and among hospital delivery patients (n = 146) was 79%. This discrepancy can be explained as most women coming for ANC or TT injection get both services (ANC & TT) in many places at the same time and women using health services are more informed than non-users.

4.2.2.3 Health worker's performance on antenatal screening activities

The health worker's perception of high risk pregnancies

The interviews with FLHS staff (n = 15) on high risk pregnancies revealed that their perception of high risk pregnancy differs somewhat from national guideline (see table 18).

Table 18: Health worker's perception of high risk pregnancies

Risk factors	Perceived as risk pregnancy by health workers (n = 15)
Age <= 19	15
Breech presentation	15
Previous CS	14
Short stature	14
Previous stillbirth	12
Primi-parity	10
Twin pregnancy	10
Previous PPH	9
Limping foot	8
Multi-parity (G4+)	5
	Perceived as emergency situation
Loss of consciousness	15
Severe headache with blurred vision	14
Bleeding per vagina during pregnancy	14

History taking and examination

From 58 cases observed, 55% of 11 essential components of history taking was enquired and 80% of 6 essential components of physical examination was done by health workers during observed consultations. Complication in previous delivery, history of previous major illness and sexually transmitted diseases symptoms were never asked. Although fundal height was not measured with a tape measure, hand palpation using abdominal landmarks was accepted as health workers were taught this way. Laboratory investigations including haemoglobin estimation, routine urine examination and test for syphilis were not done in any case (see table 19, p. 63).

Identification and correct interpretation of high risk pregnancies: An-amnestic risk factors

Although the national guideline states that women with more than 3 pregnancies should be listed as high risk pregnancy, less than 2% of multi-parity (G4+) were advised for hospital delivery. This is in line with most health workers' perceptions. Only 33% (n = 15) perceived multi-parity (G4+) as a high risk pregnancy.

All health workers (HW) perceived young age as a risk factor and 30% of women <= 19 years were advised for hospital delivery. Although nulliparity in itself is not a risk pregnancy according to the national guideline, 16% of nulliparous were advised for hospital delivery.

All health workers perceived presence of previous stillbirth as high risk pregnancy. However, only 3 out of 12 previous stillbirth documented in antenatal registers were given referral advice.

No action was taken on one woman with previous history of PPH. No data was available on previous CS or complicated delivery.

Signs identified and action taken

Maternal height was measured in three centres out of 13 centres observed. 28 women were documented as short stature, but only 7 women were advised for hospital delivery. This may be due to the fact that although most health workers (14/15) knew that short stature is a risk factor for difficult delivery, only 1 out of 15 knew the national cut off point for short stature (148 cm).

Table 19: Essential contents of history taking, physical examination and laboratory tests done during ANC (n = 58)

	% of expected performance
Contents of physical examination observed	
Fundal height	94.8
Clinical pallor	89.7
Foetal heart	87.9
Foetal presentation	87.5
Blood pressure	86.2
Height	32.7
Total % of expected performance	**80.0%**
Content of history taking asked	
Age	100.0
Marital status	100.0
Village	100.0
Parity	89.7
Number of living child	81.0
Current complaint	81.0
Stillbirth	51.7
Abortion	51.7
Complication in previous delivery	0
Previous major illness	0
STD symptoms	0
Total % of expected performance	**60.0%**
Laboratory test done	
Urine sugar and albumin	0
Blood haemoglobin	0
Test for Syphilis	0
Total % of expected performance	**0%**

All documented cases of hypertension (n = 4), breech (n = 1) and twin pregnancy (n = 1) were advised for hospital delivery. All HW perceived breech presentation as a risk factor and 67% did so for twin pregnancy.

Although all the health workers observed were able to do proper blood pressure measurement, only 8 out of 15 knew the national cut off point for high blood pressure (>= 140/90 mmHg). Although examination was done properly in most of observed consultations, there were very few documented cases for risk factors in reviewed antenatal registers. There seems to be improper documentation or the influence of observation had made better performance.

Sensitivity of the screening process

Among hospital deliveries interviews all 4 cases of twins and a case of breech presentation were not detected during ANC. The most frequent reasons for antenatal referral among hospital deliveries were weakness of the mother and anaemia.

4.2.2.4 Intervention according to risk factors and health problems identified: Referral to referral level hospital

Reasons for referral advice

From 136 antenatal exit interviews, 17.7% (n = 24) of women were advised for hospital delivery or referred to doctor's ANC. However, in their antenatal cards (n = 136) only 13.2% (n = 18) of referral advice were recorded. Reasons for referral advice given by the women and recorded at their antenatal cards are presented in table 20, p. 65.

Population based referral advice rate of high risk pregnancies

From review of antenatal registers, referral advice was given to 9.5% of first antenatal consultations (n = 1378). This would be higher at the end of ANC process. Based on different data sources (antenatal registers 9.5%, antenatal cards 13.2%, antenatal attendees 17.7%), we estimate that about 15% of women attending ANC received referral advice due to various risk factors identified during antenatal consultation. From this estimation and ANC coverage of 28%, estimated population based referral advice rate was 4.2%.

Results

Out of 146 hospital delivery cases interviewed within the 3 months' period, only 4 women were admitted as emergency cases, out of an expected 3050 deliveries at home and at FLHS from the district during the same period. From this data and the institutional delivery rate of 9.8%, the estimated emergency admission was only 0.3% of expected deliveries from the district.

Table 20: Reasons given for referral advice according to antenatal attendees and recorded in antenatal cards (n = 136)

Reasons for referral advice	Given by antenatal attendees (n = 24)	Recorded in antenatal cards (n = 18)
Previous stillbirth	4	2
Abnormal lie	3	1
Weakness	3	4
Previous difficult labour	2	1
Previous neonatal death	2	1
Swelling of hands and legs	2	3
Nulliparity	1	1
Multi-parity	1	1
Young age	1	0
Anaemia	1	2
Twin	0	1
Chest pain	0	1
HW does not tell her	4	0
Total	24	18

Referral compliance

Out of 146 maternity cases interviewed, 13.7% received referral advice during their ANC. Based on this data and hospital delivery rate of 9.8%, only 1.3% of expected deliveries from the district were actually referred as a result of ANC.

Given a population based rate of referral advice from antenatal care of 4.2%, the estimated compliance rate with antenatal referral advice was about 32%.

According to national guideline and reviewed antenatal registers, 41.5% of antenatal attendees were high risk pregnancies. They represented 11.6% of expected deliveries from the district.

The following figure 4 illustrates that antenatal care contributes very little regarding the provision of appropriate obstetric care.

Figure 4: Effectiveness of screening in pregnancy, Banke district

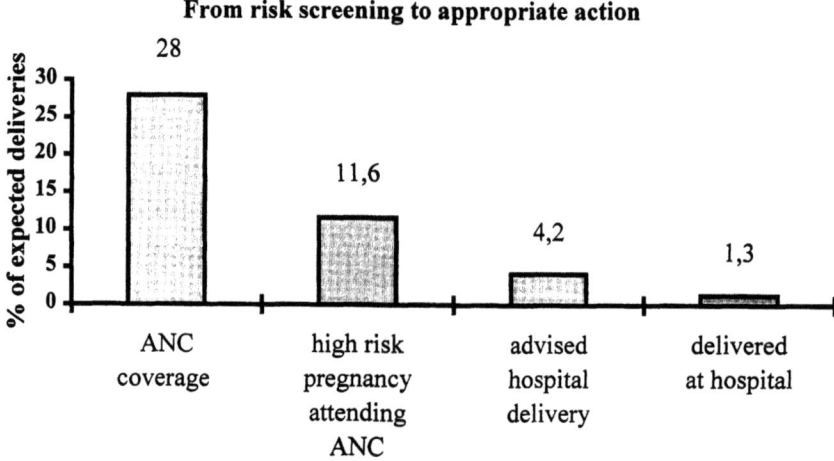

4.2.2.5 Management at referral level obstetric care

Most essential elements of obstetric care were available and fully functioning at the time of assessment. Only the partogram was not employed for continuous monitoring of labour and there was no official maternity waiting home. However, high risk cases were admitted before delivery at maternity ward. Both general and local anaesthesia were fully available at the time of assessment. Blood was almost always available from one local Red Cross association on guarantee of replacement by the relatives of the patient. There is also an intensive neonatal care unit and intensive cardiology care unit. From this findings EOC is scored as presented in table 21, p. 67.

Caesarean section can be done at both the government and the private hospital on a 24 hours basis. However, one out of 50 women scheduled for CS was

Results

referred to another centre for CS during the last 4 months due to absence of an anaesthetist.

Table 21: Availability of EOC at government hospital

Item of essential elements of obstetric care*	Scores (n/2)**
Surgical obstetrics	2
Anaesthesia	2
Medical treatment	2
Blood transfusion	2
Manual procedure and continuous monitoring of labour by qualified staff	1
Management of women at high risk	1
Family planning	2
Neonatal care	2
Total (100% = 16)	14

* WHO (1991a)
** scoring: point 2 = functioning and fully available;
point 1 = functioning but partially available;
point 0 = not available.

Care at admission, delivery and discharge

The knowledge of the hospital staff interviewed was used as a proxy indicator for the quality of care during admission, delivery and discharge. A short knowledge test on care at admission, care of normal delivery, new born care and post natal care on discharge was done with 4 staff from government hospital. (see annex 10:71-74)

The knowledge of staff about the activities they should perform on admission was 73% of expected performance (n = 4). Average knowledge of hospital staff (n = 4) on routine delivery care was 83%, routine new born care 90% and post delivery care on discharge was 80%. The partogram was not employed.

Timeliness of care

The time lapse between admission and attendance by staff and between decision for and actual performance of CS were used as indicator for timeliness of care. Out of 146 maternity interviews 22% were attended immediately at admission. 80% got attention within 10 minutes and 98% by 30 minutes.

The time needed for preparation of emergency operation (CS) was 30 minutes according to theatre staff interview. However, the average time lapse between decision for and actual performance of CS in 20 maternity cases interviewed was 4 ½ hours (range 40 minutes - 11 hours). Most of delays were due to busy obstetricians who were overloaded with first level activities.

Output related to obstetric care at referral level

Out of 1171 deliveries at the Bheri hospital CS was done in 12.5% and forceps extraction was 1%. Breech deliveries represent 1.8% and twins' 1.3%. Only 3 cases were referred to other centres.

The indication for CS was available in 54 cases of CS from both hospitals. CS was done in 35% of cases for purely foetal indication. Others were done for indications that could endanger the mother as well as the baby except in one Intra-uterine foetal death (IUFD) (see table 22, p. 69).

Coverage of high risk pregnancies at referral level

Among hospital deliveries, accumulation of high risk cases in comparison to expected frequency in the population was not observed except relatively higher cases of young age, nulliparity and bleeding. In cases of previous CS, breech presentation, hypertensive disorder in pregnancy, and multi-parity, they represented less than the expected frequency in the population (see table 23, p. 69).

Results

Table 22: Profile of CS by indication, government & private hospitals (n = 54)

Indications	Number of CS	%
Foetal distress	19	35.0
Obstructed labour	7	13.0
Abnormal presentation of foetus	7	13.0
Non-progress of labour	7	13.0
Ante-partum haemorrhage (APH)	5	9.5
Previous CS	2	3.7
Pre-eclampsia & eclampsia	2	3.7
Ruptured uterus	1	1.9
IUFD	1	1.9
Others	3	5.6
Total	54	100%

Table 23: Frequency of risk factors among hospital deliveries and pregnant women in the population, government hospital (n=1171)

Risk Factors	Expected frequency of risk factor in population %	Frequency of risk factor among hospital deliveries %	coverage of high risk pregnancies at referral level %
Nulliparity	23.0*	44.1	18.8
Young age (<=19)	18.7*	21.0	11.0
APH & PPH	3.0**	4.3	14.1
Multiple pregnancy	1.3**	1.5	11.3
Breech presentation	3.0**	2.0	6.5
Previous CS	0.9*	0.5	5.4
PET	4.7****	1.2	2.5
Multi-parity (>4)	38.6*	13.7	3.5

* = Pradhan et al. (1996)
** = UNICEF & MoH (1996)
****= WHO (1991b)

4.2.3 Outcome of maternal health care in referral level

Although there are many factors determining maternal mortality and stillbirth rates, available hospital data from the government hospital is presented as an outcome of maternal health care in Banke district. User satisfaction is presented in 4.3.

4.2.3.1 Stillbirth rate

Stillbirth (SB) rate in the government hospital was 70/1000 births. SB rate was higher among women coming from more than 30 Km distance (278/1000 births) as compared to women within 30 Km distance (67/1000 births) from the hospital. It was also higher among rural women, breech delivery, twin delivery, CS and birth weight less than 2000 gm. (See table 24, 25 & 26).

Table 24: Stillbirth rate by mode of delivery, government hospital

Mode of delivery	Number of SB	Number of births	SB rate (per 1000 births)	P value
Normal vaginal delivery	52	976	53	
CS	21	147	143	< 0.05
Breech	5	21	238	< 0.05
Twin	4	30	133	
Forceps extraction	1	12	83	

Table 25: Stillbirth rate vs. place of origin & mode of delivery among hospital deliveries, government hospital (n = 1186)

Place of origin & mode of delivery	Number of total births	Number of SB	SB rate (1000 total births)
Urban & vaginal	633	25	39
Rural & vaginal	406	37	91
Urban & CS	96	9	94
Rural & CS	51	12	235
Total	1186	83	70

Results

Table 26: SB by birth weight among vaginal delivery, Bheri zonal hospital (n = 1039)

Birth weight	Number of SB	Number of births	SB rate (per 1000 births)
>= 2500 gm	25	833	30
< 2500 gm	37	206	180
Total	62	1039	60

4.2.3.2 Maternal mortality ratio

Maternal mortality ratio among hospital delivery was 735/100,000 live births and among CS was 2380/100,000 live births.

We were able to collect delivery data by trained TBA covering 2429 deliveries in the year 1996/97 (2053/54). Stillbirth rate with trained TBA was 32/1000 total births and MMR was 576/100,000 live births.

4.2.4 Co-ordination and supervision among health workers

64% of health workers received at least one supervisory visit from district or from health post staff. 63% of health workers interviewed gave supervisory visits to other health workers or TBA.

All health workers interviewed were aware of the number of TBA in their catchment area. There is no co-ordination in terms of patient care, that is health workers are not aware of cases referred by TBA.

4.2.5 In-service training of health workers

5 out of 14 health workers interviewed had got in-service training on safe motherhood during the last one year (one health worker interviewed is a nurse student).

4.2.6 Community involvement in health care delivery

The health committee at VDC level support the FLHS in special programmes and campaigns such as the community drug programme and out reach activities.

However, there is little co-ordination in day-to-day activities of the health centres. There seems to be little co-ordination with non-governmental organisation which have health related programmes.

4.3 Determinants of maternity care services utilisation

To identify the determinants of maternity care services utilisation, both quantitative and qualitative methodology were applied. Users satisfaction was obtained from antenatal attendees. Community perspectives on modern antenatal and delivery care services were obtained by 6 focus group discussions among village women and 21 key-informant interviews.

The determinants of maternity care services utilisation will be presented as:
1. Quality of service according to service users,
2. Beliefs and practices of community regarding pregnancy and childbirth,
3. Risk perception by community regarding pregnancy and childbirth,
4. Choice of healers according to beliefs on illness aetiology, and
5. Determinants of use of modern health services in pregnancy and childbirth.

4.3.1 Quality of service according to service users

This data is derived from antenatal exit interview. The following criteria were used to assess user's view on quality of service: waiting time, reasons given for choosing this centre, reasons given for intended place of delivery, satisfaction with particular contents of antenatal care and suggestions given by users for improvement of services.

Waiting time

Average waiting time for antenatal attendees from arrival to the FLHS to her individual consultation was 90 minutes with a range of 2 minutes to 3 hours. About 33% of women complained of having to wait too long. A waiting time of more than 30 minutes was considered as long waiting time. Out of 136 women interviewed 117 (86%) were able to give approximate waiting time. The following table 27 illustrates the relationship of waiting time and complaints by attendees. Waiting time of more than 30 minutes was related with the complaint of waiting too long.

Reasons for choosing this centre

Reasons for choosing this centre, according to antenatal attendees (n = 136), were as given in the following table 27, some women gave more than one reason. 68.5% of reasons for choosing related to the service itself such as good service, nearby and free/cheap service. 18.2% were given as lack of choice.

Table 27: **Reasons given for choosing this centre for antenatal care (n = 136)**

Reasons given	Number of women giving this reason	%
Nearby to her place	60	37.7
No other place she knows	29	18.2
Free/cheap service	28	17.6
Due to good service experienced by herself or others	21	13.2
HW called her	9	5.7
Others	12	7.5

Reasons for coming to ANC

The reason given for using antenatal care services by 136 attendees were as follows. Out of 173 reasons the most frequent reasons were:
1. to know condition of baby (27%),
2. to ensure health of mother and baby (26%),
3. to know position of baby and prevent danger in delivery (19%),
4. due to problem during this pregnancy and previous delivery (11%),
5. for immunisation (10%), and
6. for getting advice and treatment (5%).

Reasons for intended hospital or home delivery

Out of 136 antenatal attendees interviewed, 70% intended to deliver at home, 18% at hospital and 12% were undecided yet. 16 women gave more than one reason for choosing the intended place. Table 28 & 29 (see p. 74) show reasons for intending hospital or home delivery.

Claimed benefits from ANC

The benefit claimed by antenatal attendees (n = 136) are as follows. 77% gave sense of safety due to the knowledge that possible problem will be identified and treated accordingly. 17% gave benefit of knowing about nutrition, cleanliness and of tetanus vaccination. 6% gave sense of safety by easier delivery and less danger in delivery. 30% claimed no benefits.

Table 28: Reasons given for intending hospital delivery by antenatal attendees (n = 25)

Reasons	Number of women giving this reason	%
Safe & good service	15	54
HW advice	9	32
Previous difficult delivery	3	11
Previous hospital delivery	1	3

Table 29: Reasons given for intending home delivery by antenatal attendees (n = 95)

Reasons	Number of women giving this reason	%
Socio-cultural reason: help from family, family member with her	35	36.8
Lack of financial resources for hospital delivery	18	19.0
Health worker/TBA will assist her at home	18	19.0
Previous delivery without problem at home	17	17.9
Family will not allow to go to hospital	8	8.4
Do not want to die in hospital	2	2.1

Patient satisfaction

Out of 136 antenatal women interviewed 81% were satisfied with the health workers' attitude towards them, 77% with the examination done by health workers, 43% with the assurance they got and 70% with the explanation they received for drug dosage.

Suggestions

Suggestion was asked from 90 ANC attendees. 49 (54%) women were not giving any suggestion and expressed that the service is OK or no idea. Suggestions given by others for improving the service are presented below.

Table 30: Suggestions given to improve services by antenatal attendees (n = 49)

Suggestions	Number of women giving particular suggestion
Free medicine	12
Doctor should come to FLHS	9
Good information and advice (counselling)	8
Less waiting time	6
Better attitude of health worker	3
Separate check up room	2
Proper examination	1

4.3.2 Beliefs and practices of community regarding pregnancy and childbirth

The following important issues emerged during the six focus group discussions conducted with a total of 56 participants: nutrition, clean delivery, physical rest, sexual behaviour and medical intervention.

Nutrition

Good nutrition such as eating green vegetables, meat and fish for the health of both mother and baby is mentioned by most of the focus groups. They try to eat good food during pregnancy and after delivery even if they were not able to eat in other time. *"It is our custom to eat good food during pregnancy"* mentioned one lady. Although they emphasised the importance of good nutrition during pregnancy, they also mentioned lack of money for buying such food: *"they eat fruits and fish which they catch"*. Food taboos during pregnancy was not encountered during the discussions, *"what ever we like and we get, we eat"*. However, food taboos was not probed in detail.

Eating extraordinary things such as mud and ashes during pregnancy is seen as a natural process and is quite common during pregnancy. They explained that the baby inside needs this: *"Because the baby of the abdomen wants mud, so it can digest mud"*.

In the Hindu community, women are not allowed to eat food immediately after delivery and allowed only after they underwent the ritual process *puja*[3] to their god. *"The mother cannot eat anything, she has to stay the whole day only with water. After puja we feed her good food"*. After delivery women said they consume good food such as meat, fish and *jaod* (beer made of honey) for the health of the baby.

Clean delivery

Personal hygiene is emphasised in most discussions during pregnancy, delivery and after delivery. They related lack of cleanliness in delivery with disease that ultimately leads to an unhealthy baby. Using clean equipment for delivery *sutkeri samagri* (delivery kit newly introduced by *Nepali* government) is seen as important and some groups are concerned about TBA who do not use *sutkeri samagri* in delivery care. The expectant women buy at the local market if they can afford money. Emphasis was also made on prevention of tetanus by personal cleanliness.

Hard working and rest

In this area two divergent concepts came up with the discussions.

Most groups mentioned the importance of rest during pregnancy. *"We stop to carry heavy things"; "If we had two jobs, we start to do only one"; "They take rest by lying in day time"*, were mentioned by focus groups.

---
[3] **Puja** = A religious ritual done to cure disease or eliminate evil things

In contrary to the emphasis on physical rest during pregnancy, there is a belief among some villagers from two focus groups that hard working before delivery will enhance easier delivery. *"If a pregnant woman works hard she sweats, baby also sweats, so the baby's head will not be big. It is easy to give birth"*, mentioned one woman from Naubasta village. *"In my time mother-in-law and other relatives thought that if I pound the rice with hand it helps the baby to come out easily. They believe that every time I pound the rice and the baby goes down. Like that baby took birth"* mentioned another woman from Paraspur village who was supported by others.

Sexual behaviour

Abstinence from sexual intercourse after 5 months of pregnancy is mentioned in some discussions, but this seems to be in the transition period from traditional to modern practice of non-abstinence.

Medical intervention

Tetanus toxoid vaccination and vitamins are perceived as important and mentioned as reasons for going to modern health services.

4.3.3 Risk perception by community regarding pregnancy and childbirth

According to the focus group discussions, there are problems perceived to be dangerous for pregnant women and the baby and which trigger care-seeking from different care givers such as home remedy, traditional healers and modern health service. These include: various pains, baby not moving, cannot give birth, baby not in position, placenta could not come out, more bleeding, fever, convulsion, white discharge of various origin, weakness due to bone melting, illness due to witch taking food (vomiting and loss of appetite) and tetanus.

4.3.4 Choice of healers according to beliefs on illness aetiology

Healers are chosen according to the beliefs on the cause of illnesses and/or perceived severity of illness. In most problems during pregnancy and delivery, women initiate treatment with a home remedy. If there is no improvement, they seek care according to the beliefs of causation of illness. Most cases are treated at home with herbal medicine (also with drugs from pharmacy) and followed by traditional or modern medicine. However, in some instances they seek care from modern health care as soon as they recognise the problem.

In the following I will present choice of healers with type of problems they encountered during pregnancy and childbirth.

Vomiting and loss of appetite in pregnancy

They believe that vomiting and loss of appetite in pregnancy is due to a witch who takes good food from the women. They seek treatment from a local traditional healer, a *guruwa*, and he performs a *jarfuk*[4] to cure the illness. However, some women buy drugs from the pharmacy for this problem. When women become more weak and cannot eat any food, they go to the hospital as a last resort.

STD-related symptoms

In case of vaginal discharge and STD-related symptoms, the choice of healer depends on diverse beliefs on explanation of causation. The following statements illustrate the diversity in beliefs on causation and health-seeking behaviour.

Some do not perceive vaginal discharge as a disease during pregnancy and seek no treatment: *"It is because of baby, it is not from others. It is called* **dhadu**[5]*"; "We get this when we are pregnant. But it is cured once we deliver baby".*

Some believe that it is due to weakness: *"It is due to weakness, if she is not eating well she gets discharge, ---- is called* **dhaat**[6]*"* explained by one woman and supported by many discussions.

The idea of white discharge being a presentation of melting bone and weakness is explained by two groups: *"melting bone cause white discharge and weakness, they go to* **guruwa**. *If they are very weak and hands and legs become swelling and pain or in fever, they go to hospital. In this situation everybody will go to hospital."*

---

[4] *Jarfuk* = Ritual ceremony performed for curing diseases with supernatural origin
[5] *Dhadu* = White discharge due to pregnancy
[6] **Dhaat** = White discharge due to weakness

The idea of getting disease due to not adhering to local rules is quite common among the community:
*"The way of transfer is if a person suffering from disease passed urine, the person who crossed by that urine gets the disease. It is called **nagan**[7], healer said it is due to evil spirit";*
"If you urinate in a place where water comes";
"If you urinate in the place where someone with disease urinated" ;
"—she get disease due to witch eyes" , explained by focus group participants. In these cases they go to the healer, who gives ***jadabhutti***[8] from the forest while he is doing the ritual. Healer gives ash and a ***bhutti***[9] to wear in neck. *"If they are really caught by evil spirit, they can be cured by this treatment".*

The idea of transmission by sexual contact is also mentioned. In these cases they seek modern medical treatment from the health service or drug retailer. *"It is contagious, from husband to wife"; "if women have more partners, she get discharge,--- called **panijane**[10]",* explained in focus groups.

Retained placenta

Retained placenta is perceived as a condition that needs hospital treatment: *"We have to go to hospital. Placenta is a poison. In village people cannot do anything".*

However, before they go to the hospital home remedy is sought in order to get rid of the placenta: *"Before that (going to hospital) they dig the ground, boil the water and put in the pit, they let her sits on the vapour of water, with the hot vapour the placenta will come out".*

Prolonged labour

There is also a divergence of beliefs about the causation of prolonged labour. Some believe that it is due to an obstructed birth canal. Treatment is sought by lubricating the birth canal to make easier delivery: *"They give her eggs and hot tea with ghee (local butter). Egg white and ghee will lubricate, so the baby comes out".*

---

[7] ***Nagan*** = White discharge caused by evil spirit
[8] ***Jadabhutti*** = Herbal medicine from traditional healer
[9] ***Bhutti*** = Necklace that prevents and defends evil spirit
[10] ***Panijane*** = White discharge due to germs

Belief in evil spirits that cause difficult delivery was also mentioned. Moreover, care from traditional healer is sought to drive out evil spirits: *"If she can't give birth, they call **guruwa** and he do **jarfuk** while saying some words and throwing rice as evil/bad things"*.

High fever

Fever during pregnancy and after delivery is considered as a condition that requires care. However, home remedy with herbal medicine or medicine from healers is applied before seeking care from modern health services: *"In house we put ginger, black pepper, chilli, sugar in hot tea and give it to the women. If she is not better, then we go to hospital"*.

4.3.5 Determinants of use of modern health services in pregnancy and childbirth

Determinants of utilisation of modern health service in care during pregnancy and childbirth are derived from 6 focus group discussions and 21 key-informant interviews.

4.3.5.1 The influence of cultural tradition on use of services
Pregnancy and delivery seen as a natural process

In this community pregnancy and delivery are considered natural processes that do not require extra medical care. All focus groups and key-informants explained that they do not seek care unless there is some problem during pregnancy and/or delivery. *"If we feel difficult then we go to hospital, otherwise everything is up to God"*, was mentioned by one lady. *"Pregnancy and delivery are considered a situation which is supposed to take it's natural course"*, explained a key-informant. *"If women are not in problem they will not go to ANC. They used to say if we don't have problem why should we go?"*.

Most women in the focus groups had a home delivery. They explained that it is their culture to deliver at home with mother-in-law or old ladies from the community, which is considered as adequate. *"If some one is going to deliver a baby, we use to call women from our own area, but she must be experienced. If she cannot deliver even with the experienced women then we take her to hospi-*

tal"; "Mother-in-law and lady relatives assist delivery which is considered as adequate".

Childbirth as a family event

The culture of childbirth with relatives around is considered as one important and ongoing culture that prevents use of hospital service even in cases of emergency. *"It has been a social custom to deliver at home with relatives"; "In delivery time all known person from the village come and all people are helping the women".*

Most mentioned that women want to deliver with relatives. Old ladies are considered as the best attendant for delivery care and most deliveries are assisted by mothers-in-law and old lady relatives.

Shyness and fear

Women's isolation and restriction to the home often prevents them from using referral level care. Fear is seen as a reason for not following referral advice. *"They are afraid to be seen by stranger people other then their relatives"; "without men we cannot go"*, was mentioned by focus groups participants and key-informants.

Shyness is also mentioned quite often by key-informants as the reason for not going to ANC and not using trained staff for delivery care. In the focus groups, some participants thought that some women even died at home because they are too shy to go to the hospital and afraid of public places: *"Because of shame they don't go to hospital and people died".*

Social status of health workers

Cultural influences play a role in the practice of modern health workers. There is a belief that one lowers one's caste by cutting the umbilical cord. Some health workers are afraid that their caste will be lowered if they cut umbilical cord in delivery care. This leads to not providing delivery care services by health workers. However, most of health workers and also TBA are not deterred by cultural beliefs in their service delivery. Some manage by asking a lower caste woman to cut the cord. *"If one cut the cord of a low caste women, we consider her as a low caste" "I ask a low caste women, she gets 100 Rupees for cutting cord".*

4.3.5.2 The influence of health service factors

Relatively new services

The reason that ANC services are started very recently in many FLHS has influenced utilisation. Moreover, this was frequently mentioned by many key-informants and focus groups as the reason that women were not informed about the presence of services: *"ANC services are very new, there was no proper service before", "before our time there was no check up of pregnant women in the village, now women are going".*

Performance of health workers

Lack of sufficiently trained health workers is also mentioned as a reason for not using modern health services. Some women were not convinced by health workers' performance or advice due to previous experiences (sensitivity of risk screening): *"She checked my whole (physical examination), I was 8 months pregnant and had to go to the hospital as the baby was in breech position. But I didn't go there, I delivered at home normally".*

Non-motivation of health workers is also blamed for non-use of health services by some key-informants.

Hospital regulations which do not consider cultural value

Difference between cultural value and hospital regulation is one reason that hinders the use of referral level care services expressed by key-informants and focus groups: *"They want to deliver with relatives around, which is Nepali culture, which is also not allowed in hospital"; "In problem we go to hospital-, but I think if there is some women around us that would be nice".*

Expensive hospital fees vs. free service by local healers

Expensive hospital services together with free or low cost services by local healers is also mentioned as a reason for non-use of referral level health care

even in cases of emergency situation. Financial inaccessibility of hospital services is mentioned by many key-informants and focus group discussions.
"We are daily wages labourers. If we go to hospital it cost high. At least we need 1000, 2000, If we do not have that much money, we could not take her to hospital. If someone can pay for us then it is OK, we could pay him in instalment".
"If there is no help we cannot go, they (mother & baby) will die at home".
"Some sell their land".

On the other hand most traditional healers do not take money for service, but for ceremonial services. ***"Guruwa** does not take money"* "*I think we go to **bhuehar**[11] because we don't have money to go to hospital"*. Financial accessibility is mentioned as an important hindering factor even for ANC which is free in many cases. *"who got money go to HP for check up and medicine. Who have not got money will stay at home whether dead or alive".*

Organisational and geographical accessibility

Inconvenient opening hours of ANC services was mentioned as reason for non-use of ANC services. *"they are very poor, they have to work the whole day in the fields, they come in their spare time"* explained a key-informant. One MCHW adjusted her opening hour according to the season, earlier in summer and monsoon season.

Although distance and transport problems were most frequent problems identified in other studies, it was found that only some key-informants and focus groups mentioned these factors as the hindrance for utilisation of health services. However, difficulty to reach hospital during monsoon was emphasised by some key-informants, but not as often as expected.

4.3.5.3 The influence of socio-economic conditions on use of service

Lack of education

From the key-informants' perspectives, who are also part of modern health services, lack of education and ignorance or not knowing the importance of ANC was the most frequent reason given for non-use of ANC service.

---
[11] ***Bhuehar*** = Traditional healer

However, some informants failed to relate this idea with service users, whether users are more educated than non-users. *"They do not know the benefits of ANC"* was described by most of key-informants as the reason for not going to ANC.

Distribution of power and property

Women's lack of power and property in the family is described as one significant hindering factor for use of referral level care which is always expensive and needs support from the family. They cannot decide for themselves even they are convinced for the need of referral level care. This idea is shared by both key-informants and focus group participants:

"Property use to be with the husband, mother-in-law, father-in-law, so women cannot do anything. They want to save money"

"Women cannot decide themselves, family (mostly mother-in-law) have to decide"

"The old people do not allow us to go to the hospital. Old people said we didn't go to hospital, we have many children, why should you go. We cannot say anything"

"My mother-in-law stopped me to go to hospital. If she (mother-in-law) could give birth at home why should I (she) have to go to the hospital?".

5 Discussion, conclusion and recommendations

In this chapter the findings of this study are critically analysed in relation to the objectives stated and the pre-existing body of knowledge in this area. Firstly, the existing health service infrastructure in terms of availability and accessibility will be discussed. This will be followed by the discussion on the actual utilisation of antenatal and obstetric care services with reasons for low utilisation. Finally, the performance of health services regarding specific components of antenatal and obstetric care, including the pathway from screening to appropriate management of high risk cases will be analysed.

5.1 The infrastructure and organisation of maternal health care services

One of the prerequisites for delivering effective health care is a favourable health care facility, which is accessible for the population in need. The HMG of Nepal has put emphasis on increasing the accessibility for the rural population to primary health care. Service delivery focuses on a network of community health care workers supported by a number of first line health services.

Although FLHS are fairly distributed throughout the district, the health infrastructure in the district is inadequate to deliver an equitable and quality health care for antenatal as well as delivery care. This is mainly due to the absence of maternity care services in many FLHS, which is attributed by the lack of female health workers and/or the lack of motivation of health workers. As most centres have only one or two rooms shared by two or more health workers, providing ANC in a more integrated way seems to be difficult in the near future. Moving services nearer to people by providing more outreach points seems to be a more promising path in this situation and community, where a woman's domain is her home and her mobility is relatively restricted.

Home delivery care was not provided by all staff who do provide ANC. Institutional delivery care service was not available in all FLHS and they are not equipped and ready to give basic EOC. Referral level care at the government hospital, as in many developing countries, is inaccessible geographically and financially, especially for the rural population.

The availability of staff, essential equipment, drugs and supplies is limited and comparable to other countries (Gilson et al. 1995). The importance of accessible and well-equipped facilities was also perceived by the community as a vital part of a health care system. The absence being regarded as poor quality of care and becomes a reason for dissatisfaction with the service and a disincentive factor for seeking care in this study as well as in other studies (Oyeledun, 1997; Thaddeus and Maine, 1994). As the hospital has to recruit local staff to overcome the excessive workload, the user fees could not cover all the expenses to buy the necessary materials and supplies that increase with complicated cases. This in turn creates a barrier for emergency cases when the financial situation of the family is difficult.

The relationship of geographical inaccessibility of services with low utilisation and high maternal deaths is well documented. There are options to overcome this problem by moving the service to the periphery or by moving the person in need nearer to the service (Thaddeus and Maine, 1994). In Banke, by moving the services through outreach points together with a number of TBA in the community, geographical accessibility to basic maternity care is enhanced and seems to be the most suitable way to improve utilisation of maternity care services. With regards to EOC, although improvements could be made with providing EOC at all the higher level FLHS, the burden cannot be solved by the health sector only. Integration and collaboration with other sectors are inevitably essential.

5.2 Utilisation of antenatal and obstetric care services in Banke district

Utilisation of health services is a precondition for fulfilling the objective of health for all by 2000 and is perceived by health planners and health care providers as an important indicator. To provide effective care, the assumption is that the community makes use of available health care services. This is not yet the case in this district. In spite of increasing utilisation of maternity care services in Banke district, coverage is still low in comparison to many developing countries (70% for ANC coverage for all developing countries) (WHO 1997).

There is concern about the low utilisation of ANC services in this district. Although there are doubts about the effectiveness of ANC in the prevention of

Discussion, conclusion and recommendations

maternal and perinatal deaths, there are many studies that relate lack of or insufficiency in ANC with avoidable maternal and perinatal deaths (Kwast, 1989; Wilkinson, 1997; Belsey and Wiest, 1993). Higher maternal mortality was observed among non-users of ANC service (Konje et al. 1990).

Concerning the coverage of ANC by individual FLHS, two interesting findings were observed. Firstly, there is diversity in utilisation of individual services and secondly, higher utilisation of lower level services. Utilisation depends on accessibility and acceptability of a service. With similar infrastructure, variation in individual service utilisation highlights the very important role of quality of care regardless of level of training. The finding that lower level services are utilised more stand in contrast to other studies that found people appreciate higher level services (Sauerborn et al. 1989). This may be due to the fact that some FLHS cover a wide area with bigger population and only SHP provides outreach programmes, allowing the pregnant women a chance to overcome the geographical barrier. Although MCHW (SHP staff) are trained only for a short period, they are from the same community, were recruited by the local village development committees and are supposed to work in the same area. All these factors contribute to better communication with the community, and the sense of "being local" motivates better than others as seen in the fact that all MCHW provide home delivery care services. Another factor could be that for a rural woman it is easier to talk to a person they know already. Moreover, when a higher level health worker does not provide service other than the lower level one, people judge them by service provided and not by training level.

The importance of early attendance and intervention according to the needs of pregnant women has been stressed by many studies (Munjanja et al. 1996; Gissler and Hemminki, 1994). Poor outcome was related with antenatal attendance later than 16 weeks in Finland (Gissler and Hemminki, 1994). The study findings in Banke may be due to the fact that communities are not aware of the importance of preventive care during pregnancy and they perceived pregnancy and childbirth as natural processes that do not need extra-care. They come only when there is a problem and when they want to confirm that the baby is well. This necessitates strengthening of community health education programmes and awareness programmes. However, one interesting finding is that most health personnel seem to think they are not responsible for this important task as they easily stated "community ignorance" as a factor that deters utilisation.

In comparison to NFHS data, trained TBA were less used than untrained for delivery care. This is in line with other studies that also found non-use of trained TBA services in other countries (Nougtara et al. 1989; Sargent, 1982). Further exploration of this finding is urgent as the national safe motherhood policy depends heavily on a network of trained TBA to provide basic home maternity care.

To prevent maternal deaths, it is necessary that women with obstetric complications are treated at the level where EOC is available. The utilisation of hospital for delivery care and for complicated cases depends on availability and accessibility of the hospital as well as the perceived quality of care by the community (Thaddeus and Maine, 1994). Professional health workers share less than 20% of expected deliveries (including hospital deliveries) with high urban rural disparity. More than 65% of deliveries were taking place at home without medically trained assistant. With this low coverage, one would expect high emergency referral cases. However, only less than 1% of women from the district was admitted for complications arising during delivery, while at least 5% would need emergency admission to the hospital because of complications arising during delivery, especially where 90% of deliveries took place at home (Rooks et al. 1989; WHO, 1994c). All these findings emphasise that in Banke district most deliveries including complicated deliveries take place outside health services without necessary care to overcome serious complications, deaths and long term disability.

One threatening finding is the use of over-the-counter drugs in pregnancy related illnesses. Using these drugs in pregnancy is frightening as many could be dangerous for the baby. Moreover, most of the users as well as the drug sellers are not aware of any side effects of drugs (Kafle and Gartoulla, 1993). Health education programmes that inform the women and their families as well as the drug sellers about dangers of irrational drug use during pregnancy would be beneficial.

5.3 Why is the utilisation of maternity care services comparatively low in Banke district?

Underlying the utilisation of health services is the assumption that the service should be easily available and accessible to the population in need. Furthermore, it should be accepted by the community so that the people in need are

Discussion, conclusion and recommendations

willing as well as able to use this service. Acceptability depends on the clients' preferences which are shaped by availability, accessibility and the perceived quality of service. Other factors include the socio-cultural surrounding which influences their preference and their previous experience with health services.

In this study, determinants of maternity care service utilisation were identified as health service factors that influence utilisation and satisfaction or non-satisfaction of service users. Another factor is the socio-cultural environment that influences utilisation, the illness perception of community and their health seeking behaviour in pregnancy and childbirth.

5.3.1 Health service factors influencing utilisation

In this district, the main health services factors that determine utilisation of antenatal and obstetric care services are identified as the following:
- Relatively few maternity care service outlets with minimal service time.
- Relatively new maternity care services in the community with little awareness of the benefits from the community.
- Negative attitude of health care provider towards community awareness.
- Lack of motivation of health workers.
- Cultural beliefs that deter service delivery.
- User un-friendly organisation of ANC services that cause dissatisfaction (long waiting time).
- Financial inaccessibility of maternity care services.
- Cultural inaccessibility of hospital services.
- Perceived poor quality of health service performance by the community.

There are relatively few maternity care service outlets available for the population. It is not only because of absence of service in many places but also due to infrequent service time. This, in addition to accessibility problems, seems to be one important reason for non-use of maternity care service.

From the provider point of view, the fact that ANC services are relatively new and were not known by the community was perceived as one reason for non-use of services. This further points out the need for strengthening community mobilisation and participation in the implementation of health care programmes. Another important point was the community not being aware of the benefits of preventive health care during pregnancy and delivery. Although it may also be related to cultural perception, one should also consider the failure to involve community in health care delivery that should be initiated from the health service part. At least the woman and her family should be involved in discussing their perceptions and make them familiar with the modern technologies of intervention and their potentially positive outcome if done appropriately and in time. When the communities are aware of the benefits of using modern health service it would also become easier to mobilise community resources as, for example, in emergency transport.

The negative attitude of health care providers on community awareness needs to change as this important community awareness should be initiated from the health service part.

The influence of cultural traditions on performance of health workers has emerged in other studies (Kowalewski, 1996). Not providing delivery care was related with cultural beliefs, for example, lowering one's caste by cutting umbilical cord, among some health workers in this district. The impact of this factor on service delivery is difficult to assess from this study. However, most health workers (especially lower level) do overcome this belief. It seems to be related with motivation of health workers. Basic motivational factors such as supportive type of supervision, in-service training and a bonus system would be beneficial for staff motivation.

User satisfaction reflects all aspects of health care and modifies their future utilisation of health service (Thaddeus and Maine, 1994; Donabedian, 1988b). According to ANC service users, the quality of care seems to be acceptable as the majority is fairly happy with the service they received including health workers' attitude, which is in contrast to other studies (Kowalewski, 1996; PMMN, 1992; Finerman, 1983). However, long waiting time, demand for higher level health personnel, better information and well-equipped facilities were the main concern of the minority of non-satisfied service users. However, there was a mixed picture on satisfaction with service among focus group participants. Complaints such as expensive service, hospital regulations that ignore their preference and lack of confidence in the service became evident.

Long waiting time has been observed as one of the unsatisfactory and unacceptable factors in many health care deliveries (Oakley, 1992; Oyeledun, 1997; Nougtara et al. 1989). Non-utilisation of health services has been related with long hours spent by the women since they are the family care takers and more and more involved in generating family income. This organisational problem could be resolved by providing frequent services with long opening hours.

Financial inaccessibility of health services is a common feature in developing countries. Expensive hospital service is a strong deterrent to the use of hospital delivery care even in the case of complications, which cost even more. This is mainly due to the absence of a functioning referral system in this district. The hospital is over-burdened with self referred cases (both antenatal and obstetric care services), while referred cases from FLHS were not given any preference from the hospital service. Improvement could be made as in Kasongo study, Zaire, where continuation of care is guaranteed if patients were referred from FLHS, in terms of fee's exemption (Dujardin et al. 1995) or earlier attendance.

Hospital regulation that fails to be culturally sensitive is seen to be an important impediment for utilisation of delivery services as in other studies (PMMN, 1992; Obermeyer, 1993). This contrasts to another study from Nepal that found traditional and modern practices coexist harmoniously at the hospital delivery room (Reissland and Burghart, 1989). This was not the case in the Nepalganj hospital. Many women in this district indicated their appreciation of being accompanied by relatives in the labour room. The positive effects of psychological support during childbirth are well documented (Enkin et al. 1995,p.191-197; Sosa et al. 1980). Consideration should therefore be made for allowing family members in the delivery room.

Ordinary people are very good in judging health services. Although not a common feature, the lack of confidence in the health worker's performance is an important finding as this could deter use of health service, especially concerning referral advice. It is also a common finding in most assessments of health service (Maine, 1997). This may be due to the one way communication (top-down) in ANC together with the low predictive value of most screening procedures. Moreover, one should also consider the training obtained by MCHW to execute all these jobs and responsibilities. They receive only three months basic training from experienced ANM who has only two years training. This indicates the necessity of in-service or on-job training to maintain and increase their knowledge. Training emphasising not only technical skills but also human communication would be helpful.

Similarly, lack of confidence in hospital service was observed. Although this was voiced only by a small number among the interviewed, this is in line with some other studies where women did not perceive hospital as a safe place (Kazmi, 1995; Oosterbaan and Barreto da Costa, 1995; Dehne et al. 1995). This may be due to the fact that women who come in desperate condition due to many delays (Thaddeus and Maine, 1994) experience a higher maternal mortality and thus give the hospital a bad reputation. However, this perception needs to be explored and community's confidence on hospital care should be restored as the hospital is the only place where women's and their babies' lives can be saved in the case of obstetric complications. Further exploration is needed whether the hospital is really not a safe place or whether this is due to the failure of the whole health system as seen in other studies (Jafarey and Korejo, 1993; Walker et al. 1986).

Although the effects of incompetent health services are widely documented for utilisation of health services, this is not the only reason. For example, in rural Tanzania, despite highly deficient health service infrastructure, coverage of ANC is still nearly 100% and institutional delivery is 40% (Oyeledun, 1997; Kowalewski, 1996; Gilson et al. 1995). There are further factors that influence utilisation of health service such as socio-cultural beliefs and practices.

5.3.2 Does socio-cultural tradition play an important role in utilisation of modern maternity care services in Banke district?

Culture in this community is in transition. Although there are widespread practices stemming from modern knowledge, many cultural beliefs influence people's perception and practices of care during pregnancy and childbirth.

The main socio-cultural factors that determine utilisation of maternity care services in Banke district were observed to be the following:

- Pregnancy and childbirth are natural processes that do not require extra medical care.
- Childbirth is a family event and women prefer to be with the family and at home.
- Cutting the umbilical cord is considered to be a low-caste activity.
- The mother-in-law is perceived to be the best birth attendant.
- Different perception of illness causation shape the health seeking behaviour.
- Women's submission in the family and their value accorded in the society.
- Women's restricted mobility.

All these factors continue to influence the health seeking behaviour as seen in 90% of deliveries taking place at home with more than 65% delivered without medically trained assistant.

The perception of pregnancy and childbirth as natural physiological events that do not require extra-care is quite common in different parts of the world including South Asia, North Africa and West Africa. Women seek care only in case of problems during pregnancy as well as in delivery (Kazmi, 1995; Auerbach, 1982; PMMN, 1992). The cultural tradition that pregnancy and childbirth should preferably be taking place in family surroundings in order to perform rituals is also a common feature in other societies (Mutambirwa, 1985; Sich, 1981). In contrast to the above studies, a relation of home delivery with perceived vulnerability of pregnancy and childbirth leading to protection with "do's" and "don't" and rituals are not came across in this community. It seems to be convenience and courtesy at home environment that leads to the preference of home delivery as seen in Morocco and Tunisia (Obermeyer, 1993). This in turn deters from use of hospital service where hospital regulations do not consider traditional preference.

The concept of 'home delivery' or 'delivery in a homely environment' in developed countries finds much support as long as the expectant women could get necessary care in case of emergency situation (Rooks et al. 1989). However, in many developing country' environments, home deliveries taking place without trained assistants can lead to a disastrous condition as there are many delays in different levels of care (Thaddeus and Maine, 1994).

One interesting finding is the belief of lowering one's caste by cutting the umbilical cord in childbirth that was also seen in other studies in Nepal (Reissland and Burghart, 1989, Schutzke 1998). Under the influence of similar culture, it would be difficult and uncomfortable for the lower caste (uneducated!) women to invite an educated, probably higher caste women for the tasks that they themselves think are polluted and low. This factor seems to be an important deterring factor for utilisation of trained assistants for delivery care as seen in the low utilisation of trained staff as well as trained TBA. This necessitates the exploration of the impact of these beliefs on the utilisation of trained assistants for delivery care as it would imply reconsideration of the policy of maternity care. Moreover, preference of mothers-in-law for birth attendants seems to be in line with non-utilisation of medically trained attendants.

In many societies, choice of health care is strongly influenced by community perception of aetiology and seriousness of illness as well as the availability of alternative care (Thaddeus and Maine, 1994). Illness is interpreted according to the patient's criteria and not by medically defined criteria. Care is sought according to the perceived cause of illness, severity and amenability by a particular care (Niraula, 1994; Stock, 1983). In this district, the perceived aetiology and health seeking behaviour is clearly demonstrated in the example of vaginal discharge in pregnancy (see result 4.3.4). Different types of care were sought according to their different perceived aetiology. This is in line with other studies that found different causes of illnesses including the idea of impurity invading the body in case of pregnancy related problems and the subsequent need to purify (Oosterbaan and Barreto da Costa, 1995; PMMN, 1992).

All these perceptions not only delay appropriate care-seeking but can also be dangerous as in steaming of the birth canal done to expel a retained placenta in this community. It would be worthwhile to explore perceived causation and health seeking behaviour for individual problems during pregnancy and childbirth so that one could incorporate this knowledge in the practice of modern medicine and planning for community health education programmes.

Culturally prescribed submission of women under elders is also a factor that influences use of both antenatal and obstetric care in this community. When women lag behind in many aspects of development and have little access to property, their ability to access health care depends highly on the decision made by her husband or elders from the family. Moreover, her value increases with the number of sons she has (Acharya, 1997). This leads to a child-centred care, ignoring women's health not only by herself and her family but also by the health services (Rosenfield and Maine, 1985). This is seen in emphasis on ANC with relative laxity about postnatal care by both the service users as well as the providers.

Although not a common observation, restriction of women's mobility is one factor that deters from use of maternity care services. This becomes obvious in case of ANC where extra-care during pregnancy is not perceived as important and the women get no approval and accompaniment from the family. Together with this factor, shyness and fear of exposing oneself to strangers deter from the use of health service even if women are convinced about the benefits.

5.4 Do preventive and promotive activities in ANC benefit antenatal attendees?

One of the most effective components of ANC is the promotion of health of the mothers and prevention and treatment of some conditions that could jeopardise both mothers' and babies' health such as anaemia, infections, hypertensive disorder of pregnancy and tetanus (Rooney, 1992). In this district, this important component of ANC is deficient in all activities including health education, counselling and prophylactics against anaemia and tetanus.

Health education and counselling

Health education is mostly given during individual antenatal consultation. Mostly the communication is one-way with the health workers instructing the women about nutrition and personal hygiene.

Information and counselling are an important component of ANC to promote the health of the women and to prevent most problems from becoming serious. It is important that health services "help people see things differently, so that they can act differently or behave more appropriately" (Pigott, 1997). This view is shared by the antenatal attendees interviewed. The importance of using this opportunity has been emphasised as ANC is the only occasion where healthy women attend the health service in many countries (McDonagh, 1996; WHO, 1994c). However, it is the most neglected part in antenatal consultations as shown in this and other studies (Oyeledun, 1997; Kowalewski, 1996). Counselling in ANC is almost non-existent in this district. Emphasis on counselling according to individual needs so that the woman could understand her situation and could have an informed choice would be one component that could be improved without further structural inputs to the health services. Moreover, consideration should be made on counselling the women together with the family decision makers including husband or mothers-in-law or elders. This would create a better opportunity for women to use necessary service as most women are not able to decide for themselves. With this aspect the need for training health workers in communication skills cannot be overemphasised.

Prevention and treatment of Anaemia

Prevention and treatment of anaemia during pregnancy is one of the effective components of ANC (Rooney, 1992). Anaemia is one of the most common illnesses in developing countries among women of reproductive age and has been found to be a co-factor for nearly half of maternal deaths in a Gambian referral hospital (Hoestermann et al. 1996). In Nepal, Iron and folate supplementation to all pregnant women was recommended (national maternity care guideline). However, this study shows that it is not yet the case in this district as shown in 4.2.2.2.

To implement a programme effectively, the assumption is that the necessary structural inputs are available. However, this was not the case as only 57% of health facilities had iron tablets in stock at the time of visit and iron/folate tablets are not supplied from the district or regional level. Moreover, one officer from UNFPA explained at the feedback session that it is not possible to supply iron tablets for all pregnant women as it would cost at least 3 million dollars per year for the whole country. This emphasises the importance of rationalisation of Iron tablets that should be included in national guidelines.

Prevention of Tetanus

Immunisation with tetanus toxoid to prevent tetanus in both mother and baby is one of the most successful preventive health care activities. Nepal has implemented the policy of a life-long coverage for all women of reproductive age by giving five consecutive doses of tetanus toxoid. Immunisation was perceived as one of the benefits of ANC and was one of the reasons for coming to ANC in this study. Integration of immunisation and ANC services, as done in many places, was impressive although officially the services were fragmented in terms of temporal availability. However, the programme needs to be improved as not only the coverage is low (TT 2 coverage 12.4% for reproductive age women, 32.6% for pregnant women[12]) but also most women were not informed about the dosage and the benefits of immunisation.

Concerning performance of health workers on preventive and promotive components of ANC, it is not satisfactory both in counselling and prevention of anaemia and tetanus. This is mainly due to the lack of infrastructure and of technique orientated training of health workers. However, there are areas for

---

[12] % women who received TT2 during their last pregnancy, NFHS 1996.

improvement such as counselling according to individual needs and risk status of the women and her family so that the women and her family have informed choices. Another would be rationalisation of available resources and drugs for the one in need. For example, oral iron supplementation could be given for clinically anaemic women, young age, grand-multiparity and multiple pregnancy, as unnecessary supplementation could even be harmful (Enkin et al. 1995, p. 29-30).

5.5 Does risk approach in ANC work in this district?

The risk approach in ANC uses a screening system that classifies women in different risk categories and allows provision of special care to those in need. Although there have been doubts about the effectiveness of the risk approach in ANC, it helps to provide a minimum level of care and attention in settings where resources are scarce (Enkin et al. 1995, p. 37-39). However, the effectiveness of this system relies on proper screening and identification, appropriate action, and proper referral system backed up by referral level hospital together with acceptable and reliable operational referral criteria.

The process of screening, identification of risk pregnancy, and referral advice

Nepal uses antenatal cards that could help the health worker in proper history taking and physical examination in ANC. However, there is no guideline for appropriate action to be taken for individual risk factors in the antenatal card as well as in the national maternity care guidelines. Moreover, the risk catalogue of the national maternity care guideline is very broad. Applying only the criteria young age (<=19) and multi-parity (G4+) more than 57% of women are classified as high risk case. In this situation, nearly all women would need referral advice for one or another reason. Therefore the ability of the guidelines to be operationalised is questionable. With the low predictive value and the low effectiveness of most screening procedures, an inflation of high risk cases could even minimise the communities' perception of the quality of health worker's performance. A re-packing of the risk catalogue is necessary in order to improve effectiveness of screening in ANC.

History taking together with height measurement, if properly done, would identify 81% of risk pregnancies from the first visit (Essex and Everett, 1977). In this study, history taking did not help the health workers to identify the risk status of the pregnant women. It is mainly for patient identification. No women observed were asked for the presence or absence of complications with previous deliveries, previous major illnesses and STD symptoms. Multi-parity, one of the risk factors according to national guidelines, was not perceived as a risk factor by many health workers. Therefore, only 2% of multiparty (G4+) were given referral advice. On the other hand, a higher percentage of young age and nulliparity (not included in risk catalogue) were advised for referral, which is also in line with the risk perception of health workers.

Good physical examination was done with most women observed in this study. Short stature is a good indicator for predicting obstructed labour if the local cut off point is applied (Dujardin et al. 1996). Almost all health workers perceived short stature as a risk factor for difficult labour. However, this did not contribute to high referral advice of identified short women. This may be because most health workers do not know the national cut off point, 148 cm.

It is well documented that if serial fundal height measurement is done by tape measure, it could identify 65% of intra-uterine growth retardation and nearly 100% of multiple pregnancy and hydramnios. There is nearly 100% sensitivity of a 'high' fundal height measurement for the prediction of multiple pregnancy (Berg and McDermott, 1996). In Nepal, fundal height was measured by using abdominal landmarks. Except for patient's satisfaction, effectiveness of this procedure is doubtful without using local reference (Walraven et al. 1995).

Abdominal palpation done in later pregnancy would prompt identification of 80-90% of mal-presentations (Berg and McDermott 1996). In this study, abdominal palpation was done properly and most health workers perceived breech presentation and twin pregnancy as risk pregnancy. However, all these aspects do not necessarily lead to the identification of high risk cases, appropriate action and accumulation of these cases in hospital as one would expect. This may be also due to under-registration and that most women attend ANC only once and probably not in their late pregnancy to detect mal-presentation and multiple pregnancy. This in one way attributed to the high stillbirth rate among breech deliveries in hospital, which in turn becomes a disincentive factor for referral advice.

Discussion, conclusion and recommendations 99

Laboratory screening tests to detect syphilis, anaemia and pre-eclampsia are one of the recommended effective interventions in ANC (Rooney, 1992). However, no facilities (HP/PHC) visited in this study were able to provide laboratory screening test. It is provided only in hospitals and private clinics. This emphasises the importance of identification of high risk cases and referral with a functioning referral system so that the high risk women could have easy access to the necessary service.

The population based referral compliance rate was very low, 1.3%. Comparing with the WHO estimates of high risk pregnancies who need essential obstetric care (15% of expected deliveries), one could estimate that less than 10% of high risk women in this district received appropriate care from the process of ANC. This necessitates exploring local risk perceptions during pregnancy and childbirth and incorporating these perceptions in the development of a risk catalogue. This would prompt not only the health workers to execute appropriate action but also the client to comply with the referral advice.

With a properly functioning risk approach in ANC, one would expect a concentration of high risk women in hospital who got advice from ANC. However, a relatively high concentration of high risk cases in hospital in comparison to expected number in the population was not observed in this study. One threatening finding is that women with previous CS as well as HDP in hospital deliveries represented less than 5% of expected similar conditions in the population. A further study that explores the fate and outcome of these pregnancies would be beneficial for future planning.

Although most health workers have enough knowledge to deliver a good quality service, basic motivational factors are lacking, such as a conducive environment and in-service or on-job training that would refresh their knowledge as well as motivate them. Supportive type of supervision, which has been started recently, is another important motivational factor and should be maintained.

Looking at above findings, one could observe that knowledge and performances do not necessarily lead to proper action in screening process of ANC. In addition, with broad risk criteria without proper guidelines for individual risk factors, the perceived risk by health worker, to some extent, influenced the action they took for identified high risk cases. Use of action orientated antenatal cards may help the health workers to interpret and execute appropriate action for identified risk pregnancies (Essex and Everett, 1977). However, one should emphasise not only the technical aspects of risk screening but also the importance of individualisation and decision according to individual status and women's preference.

Management at referral level

The government hospital provides a good comprehensive essential obstetric care service. However, the functioning referral system that links FLHS and referral level is lacking, leading to over-burdening of the referral level by first level activities. EOC was accessible for only a small number of women. Moreover, hospital mortality rate is too high and the incredibly high SB rate among CS cases cause for alarm.

The idea of having a risk approach in ANC is to make the specialised care available for the one in need, that is, essential obstetric care. This is one of the most economical approaches in delivering health care in resource-scarce countries. However, most of hospital delivery cases are urban women and are self-referred cases. High risk cases referred from ANC and emergency referred cases represent only 1.6% and 0.3% of the expected delivery from the district respectively, while at least 15% of expected deliveries will develop serious complication and at least 5% would need emergency referral during delivery especially where most deliveries take place at home.

Population based CS rate was 1.1%, with only one in ten women from rural area. Although there is a concern for CS among rural unconvinced population due to the danger of ruptured uterus with subsequent delivery (Lawson, 1972), it should be noted that about 200-250 pregnant women with their baby and family in this district are suffering or dying every year because they are not able to reach the hospital for the necessary surgery.

The high hospital mortality rates further necessitate improvement in all levels of care including the community, first line, and referral level together with a proper referral system and an improvement of the community's awareness on maternal health care.

The high stillbirth rate among CS cases was the main concern for the DMO during the feed back session. This may be due to delays in reaching the referral level and long time lapse between decision for CS and actual performance of CS. A further study that explores the relation of this time lapse and the outcome of pregnancy would be fruitful. This situation could be improved by delegating FLHS for first level activities and a functioning referral system so that the over-burdened medical doctors will have time for specialised care. Moreover, perinatal audit should be introduced to promote a change in the quality of care (Mancey-Jones and Brugha, 1997).

In summary, starting from the low coverage of ANC, low detection rate of high risk women, low referral advice rate and low compliance with referral advice, the risk approach in ANC provides very little benefit for high risk women in this district.

5.6 Conclusion

Two major issues emerge from this study. Firstly, there is an overall low utilisation of maternity care services (antenatal and obstetric care) and secondly, a low effectiveness of the service delivered. These issues are interrelated as accessibility, acceptability by the community and quality of health services are important determinants of health services utilisation. However, there are evidences that many reasons for non-use of services are beyond the immediate scope of maternal health care services:

- Maternity care coverage in Nepal is lower than many other developing countries with a similar level of infrastructure (WHO, 1997). Coverage of ANC is even low in the area near to facilities providing ANC (22% within 5 Km distance) and coverage of EOC as seen in example of CS is 2.3% for population within 10 Km distance and 0.2% for more than 10 Km distance.

- Although there are many aspects of health service deficiencies identified from this study, quality of care, both technicality and interpersonal relationship, as perceived by the users is fairly acceptable. Moreover, with similar quality of care, coverage of ANC in other countries is much higher than in Nepal, for example 95% for rural India and 98% for rural Tanzania (Oyeledun, 1997; Bhatia and Cleland, 1995).

Therefore, the conclusions will focus on the influence of the socio-cultural context of this community on their health seeking behaviour in pregnancy and childbirth followed by the specific health service aspects. Lastly, the low effectiveness of maternal health care services and its possible reasons will be addressed.

Socio-cultural factors play an important role in health service utilisation in this community

In this community, social cultural traditions, beliefs and practices play an important role in women's health seeking behaviour regarding care in pregnancy and childbirth.

The perception that pregnancy and childbirth is a normal event and it is not necessary to get extra medical care unless problems arise is prevailing in this community and influences their care of pregnancy and childbirth. Together with this and the relative restriction of women's mobility, going to ANC for a normal pregnancy is beyond consideration of the women as well as of her family and the family decision makers. The preference of familial surroundings for delivery together with hospital regulations that does not allow traditional appreciation leads to the situation where most deliveries take place at home. The caste system also plays an important role. The belief of lowering one's caste by cutting umbilical cord could be a strong factor that deters utilisation of delivery care services provided by higher caste educated trained assistants including trained TBA. Moreover, their preference of mothers-in-law for care during childbirth also in one way deters the use of trained assistant for childbirth.

In case of problems related to pregnancy and childbirth, choice of health care is influenced by their perceived cause of illness. This deters, in some extent, timely utilisation of hospital service as they seek care from different sources and modern health care becomes the last resort in many cases. These cultural traditions and beliefs determine the use of modern health services that operate within and serve the community.

Conventional deficiency of health service is impeding utilisation of health care services

Specific factors related to health services become important when the communities are in contact and familiar with these services. Both accessibility problems and poor quality of care were identified as factors deterring utilisation of health services.

The geographical accessibility problem due to few maternal health care service outlets is one important factor that impedes utilisation of ANC service (1 per

Discussion, conclusion and recommendations

12000 population for ANC). This is aggravated by user un-friendly service organisation such as infrequent service and short opening hours. However, offering outreach service gives possibility to overcome geographical inaccessibility for rural women. This seems to be highly suitable in this community where women's mobility is relatively restricted. Geographical and financial inaccessibility to hospital service is an important factor that deters utilisation of service by women in need, especially for rural population. It is impeded by the absence of a functioning referral system and the absence of basic EOC service in any FLHS.

There is a strong evidence that necessitates community mobilisation and participation in health care delivery. Blaming non-awareness of community for non-utilisation further points out the need to make health care providers responsible for this important task. The health care providers should mobilise community resources to improve health care delivery including emergency transport. Little motivation of health workers is an important aspect that shapes all aspects of health care delivery. This has contributed to providing few service outlets, user un-friendly service organisation as well as poor quality of performance, which in turn lead to lack of confidence in health services.

Low effectiveness of services for users

In this district, low quality of care was observed in both antenatal and obstetric care service. This often leads to lack of confidence on service from the community. The question arising here is "if the service quality is low, what would be its impact on the users' health?"

The potentials of both preventive and promotive activities in ANC were not fully utilised. This is related with inadequate infrastructure as well as poor performance of health workers. Poor performance of health workers, including technicality and interpersonal relationship, together with an inflated national risk catalogue often lead to non-functioning of the risk approach in ANC. Unpacking the national risk catalogue together with a clear referral guideline for individual risk factor is necessary. However, counselling emphasis on individual risk status of the women and their preference is important, which should be done in the presence of the woman as well as her family members (decision maker).

Although the hospital provides a comprehensive EOC for the district, its effectiveness is questionable. It is unacceptable that the stillbirth rate among CS and breech delivery cases is very high and the time lapse between the decision for CS and the actual performance of CS is too long. Delegation of first level activities to FLHS is necessary to improve accessibility as well as the quality of hospital EOC service. Moreover, perinatal audit should be introduced.

This study leads to the conclusion that the maternal health care services in Banke district are far behind of what is feasible in any poor and remote place in developing countries. This together with the socio-cultural context in which these services operate play important roles in the utilisation of antenatal and obstetric care services.

5.7 Recommendations

Community Level

- Mobilisation of community and involvement of community in health care should be emphasised. This important task should be initiated from the health services, particularly FLHS. Community awareness should be started with involvement of community in health care delivery. Firstly involvement of family members in the care of pregnancy and delivery by counselling the women together with her family members is highly recommended. This will also enhance use of service (EOC) as women are not the household decision makers. Awareness should also include dangers of irrational drug use during pregnancy. Community resources should be mobilised in order to organise emergency transport.

At FLHS and district level

- Accessibility of antenatal and obstetric care needs to be increased. This could be ensured by:
    filling all post of health workers and reallocation to their own post,
    providing frequent services with longer opening hours by all FLHS and offering outreach points by all FLHS.
- For the rural population, accessibility of EOC needs to be increased. This needs re-organisation of health service by:
    delegation of first level activities to FLHS,

upgrading capability of higher level FLHS in basic EOC, and a functioning referral system that ensures continuation of care.
- Perinatal audit is highly recommended in order to improve referral level care.
- Motivation of health workers should be by any means emphasised. Supportive type of supervision that has been started should be maintained. There should be at least once a year in-service or on-the-job training to refresh their knowledge. Training should include not only technical aspects, but also interpersonal relation skills. A bonus system should also be considered.
- Collaboration with other sectors is necessary to ensure accessibility of EOC.

At national level

- Reassessing the risk catalogue is necessary. The number of risk factors and their cut off point should be reconsidered. By doing so, community's risk perception should be consulted.
- A clear and distinct guideline for antenatal and delivery care should be developed from the national level and distributed to all FLHS. Contradictions of the guideline with the country specific situation should be revisited (dispensing Iron tablets to clinically anaemic women rather than to all pregnant women).

Further studies

- A further study that relates time lapse between decision for CS and actual performance of CS to the outcome of pregnancy would be fruitful to confirm the impression of this study.
- A further in-depth study that explores community's perception of illness causation in pregnancy and childbirth and their health seeking behaviour would be beneficial in planning of community awareness programme.
- An intervention study that allows adaptation of cultural traditions into modern medicine would be beneficial in order to overcome cultural inhibitions of health service utilisation. For example, allowing family members at the delivery room could be tested.

- An in-depth study that explores the impact of the cultural beliefs, for example "lowering caste by cutting umbilical cord", on the utilisation and delivery of maternity care services this community (transition from traditional to modern practice). This would be beneficial to improve utilisation and the quality of maternity care services.

Bibliography

Acharya M (1997)
Gender equality and empowerment of women: A status report submitted to UNFPA. Carts Secretarial Services, Thapathali, Kathmandu, Nepal.

Adeyi O, Morrow RH (1996)
Concepts and methods for assessing the quality of essential obstetric care. International Journal of Health planning and Management 11:119-134

Akalin MZ, Maine D, de Francisco A, Vaughan R (1997)
Why perinatal mortality can not be a proxy for maternal mortality. Stud Fam Plann 28:330-335

Annis S (1981)
Physical access and utilization of health services in rural Guatemala. Soc Sci Med 15 D:515-523

Auerbach LS (1982)
Childbirth in Tunisia: Implications of a decision-making model. Soc Sci Med 16:1499-1506

Bamisaiye A, Ransome Kuti O, Famurewa A A (1986)
Waiting time and its impact on service acceptability and coverage at an MCH clinic in Lagos, Nigeria. J Trop Pediatr 32:158-161

Belghiti A, De Brouwere V, Kegels G, Van Lerberghe W (1998)
Monitoring unmet obstetric need at district level in Morocco. Tropical Medicine and International Health 3 (7): 584-591

Belsey MA, Wiest A (1993)
An assessment of maternal and child health and family planning services- Report of an WHO expert committee. MCH/EC/WP/93.12

Berg CJ, McDermott JC (1996)
Fundal Height Measurement. In: Wildschut HIJ, Weiner CP, Peters TJ (eds) When to screen in obstetrics and gynecology. Saunders, London, pp 133-145

Bergström S, da Luz Vaz M (1992)
Mozambique - delegation of responsibility in the area of maternal care. Int J Gynecol Obstet 38:37-40

Bhatia JC, Cleland J (1995)
Determinants of maternal care in a region of South India. Health Transition Review 5:127-142

Bhatia S (1981)
Traditional child birth practices: Implication for a rural MCH programme. Stud Fam Plann 12:66-75

Bobadilla JL (1992)
Evaluation of maternal health programs: approaches, methods and indicators. Int J Gynecol Obstet 38: S 67-73

Campanella K, Korbin JE, Acheson L (1993)
Pregnancy and childbirth among the Amish. Soc Sci Med 37:333-342

Campbell M, Sham ZA (1995)
Sudan: situational analysis of maternal health in Bara district, North Kordofan. World Health Statistic Quarterly 48:60-65

Campbell O, Filippi VGA, Koblinsky MA, Marshall T, Mortimer J, Pittrof R, Ronsmans C, Williams L (1997)
Lessons learnt: a decade of measuring the impact of safe motherhood programmes. London School of Hygiene and Tropical medicine, London.

Csete J (1993)
Health seeking behaviour of Rwandan women. Soc Sci Med 37:1285-1292

Dehne KL, Wacker J, Cowley J (1995)
Training birth attendants in the Sahel. World Health Forum 16:415-419

Donabedian A (1981)
Criteria, norms and standards of quality: what do they mean? Am J Public Health 71:409-412

Donabedian A (1988a)
The quality of care - How can it be assessed? J Am Med Ass 260:1743-1748

Donabedian A (1988b)
Quality assessment and assurance: Unity of purpose, diversity of means. Inquiry 25:173-192

Donabedian A (1990)
The seven pillars of quality. Arch Pathol Lab Med 114:1115-1118

Dujardin B, Clarysse G, Criel B, De Brouwere V, Wangata N (1995)
The strategy of risk approach in antenatal care: evaluation of the referral compliance. Soc Sci Med 40:529-535

Dujardin B, Van Cutsem R, Lambrechts T (1996)
The value of maternal height as a risk factor of dystocia: a meta-analysis. Tropical medicine and International Health 1:510-521

Egunjobi L (1983)
Factors influencing choice of hospitals: a case study of the Northern part of Oyo state, Nigeria. Soc Sci Med 17:585-589

Enkin M, Keirse MJNC, Renfrew M (1995)
A guide to effective care in pregnancy and childbirth (2nd edition).
Oxford University Press inc. New York.

Essex BJ, Everett VJ (1977)
Use of an action-oriented record card for antenatal screening. Tropical Doctor 7:134-138

Feuerstein MT (1993)
Turning the tide: safe motherhood, a district action manual. MacMillan Press Ltd, London

Finerman RD (1983)
Experience and expectation: conflict and change in traditional family health care among Quichua of Saraguro. Soc Sci Med 17:1291-1298

Gadalla S, Fortney JA, Saleh S, Kane T, Potts M (1987)
Maternal mortality in Egypt. J Trop Pediatr 33:11-13

Garner P, Thomason J, Donaldson D (1990)
Quality assessment of health facilities in rural Papua New guinea. Health Policy and Planning 5:49-59

Gilson L, Magomi Ma, Mkangaa E (1995)
The structural quality of Tanzania primary health facilities. Bull World Health Organ 73:105-114

Gissler M, Hemminki E (1994)
Amount of antenatal care and infant outcome. Eur J Obstet Gynecol Reprod Biol 56:9-14

Graham WJ, Airey P (1987)
Measuring maternal mortality: sense and sensitivity. Health Policy and Planning 2:323-333

Greenwood AM, Greenwood BM, Bradley AK, Williams K, Shenton FC, Tulloch S, Byass P, Oldfield FSJ (1987)
A prospective survey of the outcome of pregnancy in a rural area of the Gambia. Bull World Health Organ 65:635-643

Hall MH, Chng PK, MacGillivray I (1980)
Is routine antenatal care worth while? The Lancet 2(8185):78-80

Hoestermann CFL, Ogbaselassie G, Wacker J, Bastert G (1996)
Maternal mortality in the main referral hospital in The Gambia, West Africa. Tropical Medicine and International Health 1:710-717

Ityavyar DA (1984)
A traditional midwife practice: Sokoto state, Nigeria. Soc Sci Med 18:497-501

Jafarey SN, Korejo R (1993)
Mothers brought dead: An inquiry into causes of delay. Soc Sci Med 36:371-372

Jahn A, Kowalewski M (1998)
The risk approach in antenatal care: pitfalls of a global strategy. Curare 15/98: 195-210

Jahn A, Kowalewski M, Kimatta SS (1998)
Obstetric care in Southern Tanzania: Does it reach those in need? Tropical Medicine and International Health (in press).

Kafle KK, Gartoulla RP (1993)
Self-medication and its impact on essential drugs schemes in Nepal. WHO/DAP/93.10

Kaunitz AM, Spence C, Danielson TS, Rochat RW, Grimes DA (1984)
Perinatal and maternal mortality in a religious group avoiding obstetric care.
Am J Obstet Gynecol 150:826-831

Kazmi S (1995)
Pakistan: consumer satisfaction and dissatisfaction with maternal and child health services. World Health Statistic Quarterly 48:55-59

Kielmann A, Janovsky K, Annett H (1991)
Assessing district health needs, services and system: protocols for rapid data collection and analysis. The MacMillan Press Ltd, London & Besingstoke

Kirkwood BR (1988)
Essentials of medical statistics. Blackwell Scientific Publications, Oxford

Kloos H, Etea A, Degefa A, Aga H, Solomon B, Abera K, Abegaz A, Belemo G (1987)
Illness and health behaviour in Addis Ababa and rural central Ethiopia. Soc Sci Med 25:1003-1019

Konje JC, Odukoya OA, Ladipo OA (1990)
Ruptured uterus in Ibadan- A twelve year review. Int J Gynecol Obstet 32:207-213

Kowalewski M (1996)
Antenatal referral practices and determinants of parturient compliance with referral advice. MSc thesis, Community Health and health Management in Developing Countries, Heidelberg University.

Kowalewski M, Tautz S, Löhken S, Jahn A (1998)
Community perspective of problems in pregnancy and childbirth.
Curare 15/98: 181-193

Kowalewski M, Jahn A, Kimatta SS, Kisimbo D (1998)
Why do at-risk mothers fail to reach referral level? Barriers beyond distance and cost. Health Transition Review (in press)

Kwast BE (1989)
Maternal mortality: levels, causes and promising interventions. J Biosoc Sci 10:51-67

Lamb WH, Lamb CM, Foord FA, Whitehead RG (1984)
Changes in maternal and child mortality rates in three isolated Gambian villages over ten years. The Lancet October 2(8408):912-914

Lawson J (1972)
The place of Caesarean section in developing countries. Tropical Doctor 2: 30-32

Lindmark G, Cnattingius S (1991)
The scientific basis of antenatal care. Acta Obstetricia et Gynecologica Scandinavica 70:105-109

Maier B, Görgen R, Kielmann AA, et al (1994)
Assessment of the district health system: using qualitative methods. The MacMillan Press Ltd, London & Besingstoke

Maine D (1991)
Safe motherhood programs: options and issues. Columbia university, New York

Maine D (1997)
Lessons for program design from the prevention of maternal mortality projects. Int J Gynecol Obstet 59 (2):S259-65

Maine D, Akalin MZ, Chakraborty J, Fransisco A, Strong M (1996)
Why did maternal mortality decline in Matlab? Stud Fam Plann 27:179-187

Malone MI (1980)
The quality of care in an antenatal clinic in Kenya. East Afr Med J 57:86-96

Mancey-Jones M, Brugha RF (1997)
Using perinatal audit to promote change: a review. Health Policy and Planning 12:183-192

McCarthy J (1997)
The conceptual framework of the prevention of maternal mortality network. Int J Gynecol Obstet 59 Suppl 2:S15-21

McCarthy J, Maine D (1992)
A framework for analyzing the determinants of maternal mortality. Stud Fam Plann 23:23-33

McDonagh M (1996)
Is antenatal care effective in reducing maternal morbidity and mortality?
Health Policy and Planning 11:1-15

Montoya-Aguilar C (1994)
Measuring the performance of hospitals and health centres.
WHO/SHS/DHS/94.2.

Montoya-Aguilar C, Marin-Lira MA (1986)
International equity in coverage of primary health care: Examples from developing countries. World Health Statistic Quarterly 39:336-344

Munjanja SP, Lindmark G, Nyström L (1996)
Randomised controlled trial of reduced-visits programme of antenatal care in Harare, Zimbabwe.
The Lancet 348:364-369

Mutambirwa J (1985)
Pregnancy, childbirth, mother and child care among the indigenous people of Zimbabwe. Int J Gynecol Obstet 23:275-285

Niraula BB (1994)
Use of health services in hill villages in central Nepal. Health Transition Review 4:151-166

Nougtara A, Sauerborn R, Oepen C, Diesfeld HJ (1989)
Assessment of MCH services offered by professional and community health workers in the district of Solenzo, Burkina Faso. I. Utilization of MCH services. J Trop Pediatr 35:2-9

Oakley A (1992)
Perspectives of users of the services. Int J Technol Assess Health Care 8 Suppl 1:112-122

Obermeyer CM (1993)
Culture, maternal health care, and women's status: a comparison of Morocco and Tunisia. Stud Fam Plann 24:354-365

Okafor CB (1991)
Availability and use of services for maternal and child health care in rural Nigeria. Int J Gynecol Obstet 34:331-346

Okafor CB, Rizzuto RR (1994)
Women's and health-care providers' views of maternal practices and services in rural Nigeria. Stud Fam Plann 25:353-361

Oosterbaan MM, Barreto da Costa MV (1995)
Guinea-Bissau: what women know about risk- an anthropological study. World Health Statistic Quarterly 48:39-48

Oyeledun B (1997)
Assessment of the quality of antenatal and obstetric care in first line health facilities in Lindi Region; Southern Tanzania. M.Sc. thesis, Community Health and health Management in Developing Countries, Heidelberg University.

Patton MQ (1990)
Qualitative evaluation and research methods (Second edition). Sage publications, London

Peters DH, Becker S (1991)
Quality of care assessment of public and private outpatient clinics in metro Cebu, the Philippines. International Journal of Health planning and Management 6:273-286

Pigott B (1997)
Orientation on safe motherhood for district programme managers (speech, Safe Motherhood day, 1997). Resident Representative, WHO, Nepal.

Pradhan A, Aryal RH, Regmi G, Ban B, Govindasamy P (1996)
Nepal Family Health Survey, Kathmandu, Nepal.

Ramji D (1997)
Personal communication.

Razum O (1994)
Improving service quality through action research: as applied in the Expended Programme on Immunization (EPI), in Medizin in Entwicklungsländern (eds) Diesfeld HJ. Peter Lang GmbH, Europäischer Verlag der Wissensctaften, Frankfurt am Main.

Reissland N, Burghart R (1989)
Active patients: the integration of modern and traditional obstetric practices in Nepal. Soc Sci Med 29(1):43-52

Bibliography

Rizvi T (1994).
TBA training project: in maternal and infant mortality; policy and interventions. Report of an international workshop at the Aga Khan University, February 7-9.

Rochat RW (1981)
Maternal mortality in the United States of America. World Health Statistic Quarterly 34:2-8

Roemer MI, Montoya-Aquilar C (1988)
Quality assessment and assurance in primary health care. WHO Offset Publication No. 105

Ronsman C, Vanneste AM, Chakraborty J, van Ginneken J (1997)
Decline in maternal mortality in Matlab, Bangladesh: a cautionary tale. The Lancet 350:1810-1814

Rooks JP, Weatherby NL, Ernst EKM, Stapleton S, Rosen D, Rosenfield A (1989)
Outcomes of care in birth centers: The national birth center study. N Engl J Med 321:1804-1811

Rooney C (1992)
Antenatal care and maternal health: How effective is it? WHO/MSM/92.4, Geneva

Rosenfield A, Maine D (1985)
Maternal mortality- A neglected tragedy: Where is M in MCH? The Lancet 2(8446):83-85

Royston E, Armstrong S (1989)
Preventing Maternal Deaths. WHO, Geneva

Samai O, Sengeh P (1997)
Facilitating emergency obstetric care through transportation and communication, Bo, Sierra Leone. The Bo prevention of maternal mortality team. Int J Gynecol Obstet 59 Suppl 2:S157-64

Sargent C (1982)
The implication of role expectations for birth assistance among Bariba women. Soc Sci Med 16:1483-1489

Sauerborn R, Nougtara A, Sorgho G, Tiebelesse L, Diesfeld HJ (1989)
Assessment of MCH services in the district of Solenzo; Burkina Faso. II.
Acceptability. J Trop Pediatr 35:10-13

Sauerborn R, Reerink IH (1996)
Quality of primary health care in developing countries: Recent experience
and future directions. International Journal for Quality of care 8, 2:131-139

Schutzte M (1997)
Personal communication.

Sich D (1981)
Traditional concepts and customs on pregnancy, birth and postpartum period
in rural Korea. Soc Sci Med 15 B:65-69

Sich D (1988)
Child bearing in Korea. Soc Sci Med 27:497-504

Smith JB, Lakhey B, Thapa S, Rajbhandari S, Neupane S (1996)
Maternal morbidity among women admitted for delivery at a public hospital
in Kathmandu. Journal of the Nepal Medical Association 34:132-140

Sosa R, Kennell J, Klaus M, Robertson S, Urrutia J (1980)
The Effect of a supportive companion on perinatal problems, length of
labour, and mother-infant interaction. N Engl J Med 303:597-600

Srinivasa DK, Danabalan M, Rangachari R (1982)
Method to assess quality of services in antenatal clinics of primary health
centres. Indian J Med Res 76:458-466

Starrs A (1987)
Preventing the tragedy of maternal deaths: A report on the International Safe
Motherhood Conference, Nairobi, Kenya

Steinmann JP and Ramji D (1996)
Beneficiary assessment of health care services (grey literature).

Stock R (1983)
Distance and the utilization of health facilities in rural Nigeria. Soc Sci Med
17:563-570

Bibliography

Taylor JE, Rooth G, Kessel E (1992)
Workshop on obstetric and maternity care, Singapore, Sept. 1991. Int J Gynecol Obstet 38:41-44

Thaddeus SA, Maine D (1994)
Too far to walk: maternal mortality in context. Soc Sci Med 38:1091-1110

PMMN (1992)
Barrier to treatment of obstetric emergencies in rural communities of West Africa. Stud Fam Plann 23:279-291

PMMN (1995)
Situation analysis of emergency obstetric care: examples from eleven operations research projects in west Africa. Soc Sci Med 40:657-667

Tinker A, Koblinsky MA (1993)
Making motherhood safe. World Bank, Washington.

UNICEF, MoH (1996)
National maternity care guidelines. FHD/MoH, Nepal & UNICEF, Kathmandu, Nepal.

van Lerberghe W, Pangu K, van den Broek N (1988)
Obstetrical interventions and health centre coverage: A spatial analysis of routine data for evaluation. Health Policy and Planning 3:308-314

Villar J, Bergsjo P (1997)
Scientific basis for the content of routine antenatal care. Acta Obstetricia et Gynecologica Scandinavica 76:1-14

Voorhoeve AM, Kars C, van Ginneken JK (1984)
Modern and traditional antenatal and delivery care. In: van Ginneken JK, Muller AS, Muller AS (Ed) Maternal and Child Health in Rural Kenya - An Epidemiological Study. Croom Helm and African Medical Research Foundation, London and Nairobi, pp 309-322

Walker GJ, McCaw AM, Ashley DEC, Bernard GW (1986)
Maternal mortality in Jamaica. The Lancet 1(8479):486-488

Walraven GE, Mkanje RJ, van Dongen PW, van Roosmalen J, Dolmans WM (1995)
The development of a local symphysis-fundal height chart in a rural area of Tanzania. Eur J Obstet Gynecol Reprod Biol 60:149-152

WHO (1978)
Risk approach for maternal and child health care: A managerial strategy to improve the coverage and quality of maternal and child health/family planning services based on the measurement of individual and community risk.
WHO offset publication 38.

WHO (1991a)
Essential elements of obstetric care at first referral level. The MacMillan Press Ltd. London, Basigstoke

WHO (1991b)
Hypertensive disorders of pregnancy: Report of a WHO/MCH inter-regional collaborative study. WHO/MCH/91.4.

WHO (1994a)
Indicators to monitor maternal health goals. WHO/FHE/MSM/94.14

WHO (1994b)
Care of mother and baby at the health centre: a practical guide. WHO/FHE/MSM/94.2.

WHO (1994c)
Mother-Baby-Package: Implementing safe motherhood in countries. WHO/FHE/MSM/94.11.

WHO (1996)
New estimates of maternal mortality. Weekly Epidemiological Record 71:97-104

WHO (1997)
Coverage of maternity care: A listening of available information. Fourth Edition

Wilkinson D (1997)
Reducing perinatal mortality in developing countries. Health Policy and Planning 12:161-165

Bibliography

Winikoff B (1995)
Is the risk approach effective in maternal care? Safe Motherhood News Letter 18:12

World Bank (1997)
World Bank report, 1997: The state in a changing world. Oxford University press.

Annexes

List of Annexes and maps

Number	Title	Page
Annex 1a	Map of Nepal	122
Annex 1b	Map of Banke district with selected health facilities	123
Annex 2a	Checklist for antenatal register	124
Annex 2b	Checklist for birth register	125-26
Annex 3a	Checklist for equipment, drugs and consumable (FLHS)	127-28
Annex 3b	Checklist for equipment, drugs and consumable (Hospital)	129
Annex 4	Checklist for observation of health worker performance	130
Annex 5	Guideline for health worker interview	131-34
Annex 6	Questionnaire for antenatal exit interview	135-38
Annex 7	Questionnaire for hospital maternity care interview	139-41
Annex 8	Guideline for focus group discussion	142
Annex 9	Guideline for key-informant interview	142
Annex 10	List of indicators to assess antenatal and obstetric care services at district level	143-56

Annex 1a: Map of Nepal

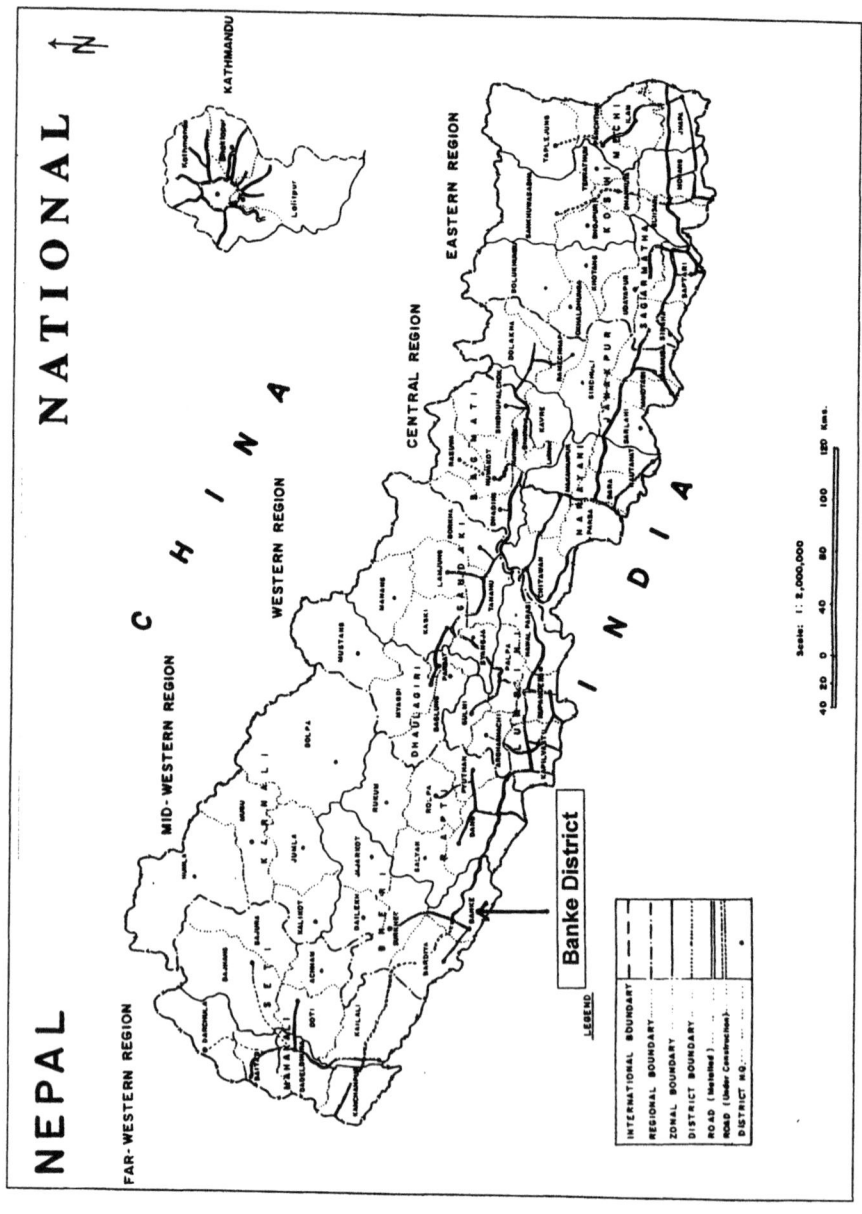

Annex 1b: Map of Banke district with selected health facilities

Bankatwa PHC	3
Belahari SHP	6
Belbhar SHP	7
Betahani SHP	8
Holiya SHP	15
KanchanapurHP	20
Kohalpur SHP	25
Kamdi SHP	19
Manikapur SHP	28
Nepalganj HP	30
Naubasta SHP	32
Paraspur SHP	33
Samsherganj HP	42
Sonpur HP	44

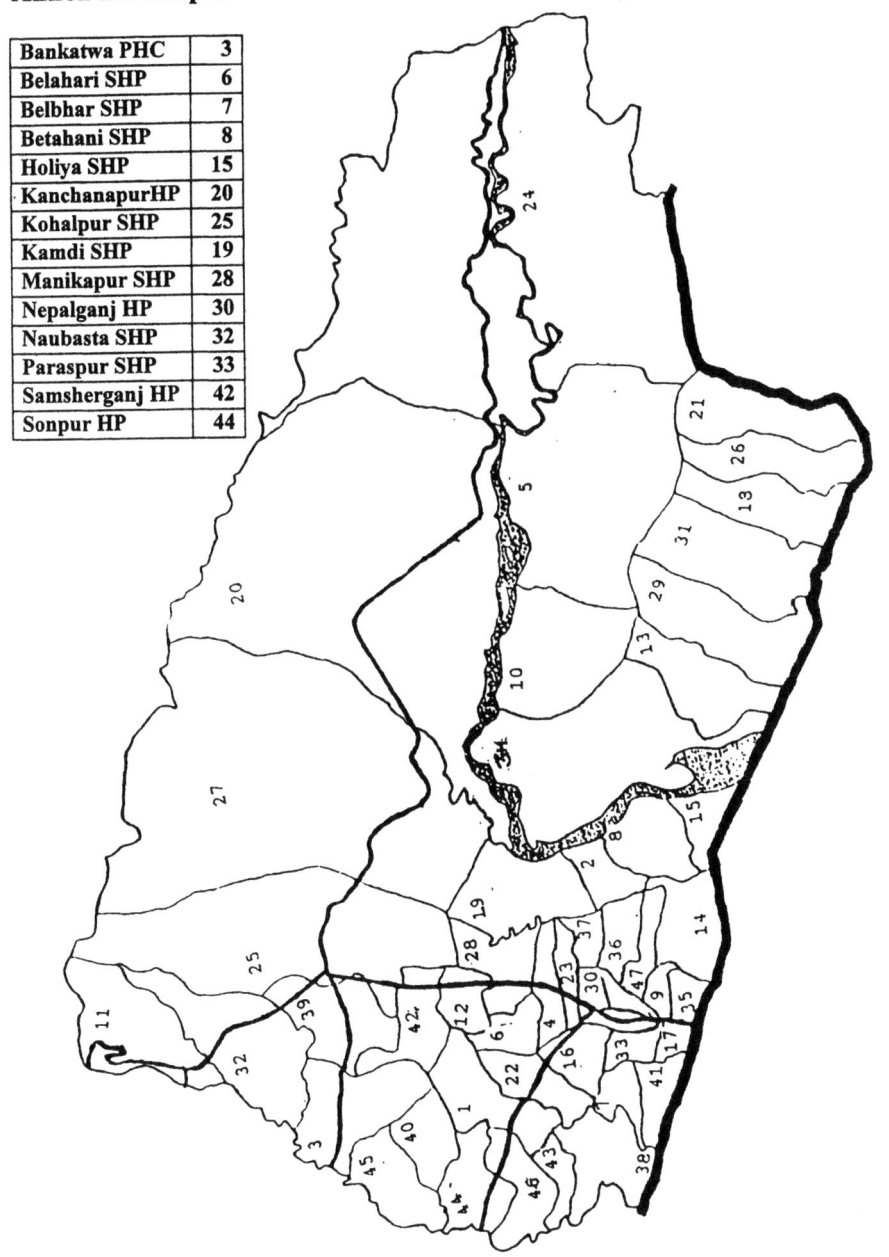

Annex 2a: Checklist for antenatal register
PHC/HP/Hospital (name) _____

Total no. of AN visit			identified/ recorded	Referral advice
number of visit		Risk factor		
1st visit		H/O still birth		
2nd visit		H/O difficult labour		
3+ visit		H/O PPH		
		<=19 year		
Religion	H= Others=	primi		
	M=	G 4+		
Age		short stature		
<= 19		high BP		
20-34		twin		
>=35		breech		
Gestation 1		anaemia		
2		oedema		
3		social reason		
4		others		
5				
6		Village (distance)		
7				
8				
9				
10 & >				
Fundal height at first visit (in weeks)				
<= 20				
21-35				
>= 36				
Contents of ANC done/recorded				
Height				
BP				
Presentation				
Lab. Test				

Annex 2b: Checklist for birth register

total number of delivery in the month of _____				
total birth				
alive				
Distance from the hospital				
<= 5 Km				
6-10 Km				
11-20 Km				
21- 30 Km				
31-60 Km				
> 60 Km				
Gestation				
	1		6	
	2		7	
	3		8	
	4		9	
	5		10 & >	
Age	<15			
	16-19			
	20-29			
	30-39			
	>=40			
Still birth	< 5 Km	6-30 Km	>30 Km	
< 2000 gm				
< 2500 gm				
twin				
breech				
CS				

Referred Cases	urban	rural
antenatally		
intrapatum		
distance < 10 km		
11-30 km		
31-60 km		
> 60 km		
risk factors		
primipara	age <=19	1+age > 35
multip 4+	Ho >2 abortion	Ho SB
multip 6+	anaemia	unmarried
breech	twin	HDP
prolonged labour	Ho PPH	
number of sepsis after normal delivery at hospital (T > 40 C x 24 hours)		
total number of CS (hospital)	urban	rural
emergency		
planned		
indications		
total number of women referred for CS from this hospital to others		
total number of operative delivery other than CS		
total maternal death from hospital		
maternal death after CS (hospital)		
total admission of ectopic pregnancies		
total admission of APH		
total admission of PPH		
total admission of obstructed/prolonged labour		
total admission of eclampsia		
total admission of sepsis (Temp > 40 degree celcius x 2 days)		
total number of days without available blood transfusion/year		

Annexes

Annex 3a: Checklist for equipment, drugs and consumable, FLHS

Name of FLHS _____

	Facility and Equipment	absent (0)	not functioning(1)	functioning (2)
1	ANC room with privacy			
2	examination bed			
3	sphygnomanometer			
4	stetoscope			
5	foetoscope			
6	tape measure			
7	for heigth measurement			
8	thermometer			
9	ANC cards			
10	standardised ANC register			
11	technical guideline for ANC			
	Total			
	DELIVERY CARE			
1	delivery room with privacy			
2	light in delivery room			
3	running water source			
4	delivery bed			
5	mucous extractor for			
6	infant weighing scale			
7	set for perineal repair			
8	urinary catheter			
9	sphygnomanometer			
10	stetoscope			
11	foetoscope			
12	thermometer			
13	standardised birth register			
14	technical guideline for			
	Total			

	Drugs and Consumable	absent (0)	present (1)	
1	chloroquine (oral)			
2	ferrous sulphate (oral)			
3	folic acid (oral)			
4	paracetamol or aspirin (oral)			
5	contraceptive pills			
6	TT (inj)			
7	ergotmetrine (inj)			
8	iv fluid for replacement			
9	iv set line			
10	sterile syringes & needles			
11	sterile gloves			
12	antihypertensive drugs (oral)			
13	local anaesthetics (inj)			
14	silver nitrate (or antibiotics)			
	Total			

Annex 3b: Checklist for equipment, drugs and consumable (hospital)

in labour room: score = n/22	absent (score=0)	non-functioning (score=1)	functioning (scroe=2)
1. vacuum extractor			
2. forceps			
3. adult ambulatory bag			
4. new born ambulatory bag			
5. heated place for new born resuscitation			
6. set for perineal repair			
7. iv fluid			
8. iv set			
9. oxytocin			
10. partograph form			
11. standardise birth register			
in theatre: score = n/22			
1. oxygene			
2. morphine or pethidine			
3. anaesthetic agent (e.g. ketamine, GA)			
4. iv fluid			
5. iv set			
6. oxytocin			
7. adult ambulatory bag			
8. new born ambulatory bag			
9. heated place for new born resuscitation			
10. suction machine			
11. standardised operation register			
Total			

Annex 4: Checklist for observation of health worker performance

Place & date

Case number	1	2	3	4	5
starting time					
Months of pregnancy					
number of visit					
Does the health worker ask the women the followings?					
1. age					
2. marital status					
3. village					
4. parity					
5. living child					
6. abortions					
7. stillbirths					
8. previous delivery complication					
9. previous major disease					
10. current complaint					
11. STD symptoms					
Does the health worker talk about the followings with the women					
1. personal hygiene					
2. nutrition					
3. when to seek medical care					
4. preparation for delivery					
5. family planning					
6. give assurance about pregnancy					
Completeness of examination					
1. height measurement					
2. check clinical pallor					
3. check oedema					
4. check BP					
5. check presentation					
6. check FHS					
Lab. examination					
1. Urine albumin					
2. Urine sugar					
3. Blood Hb%					
4. VDRL test					
ending time					

Annexes

Annex 5: Guideline for health worker interview

Explanation of the study aim: the importance of delivering quality care in pregnancy and childbirth. To find ways to improve the existing services. Assuring confidentiality.

Date of interview: .... Date/month/year |___|___|___|	
Place of interview:	
1. Qualification of health worker:	
2. Can you speak local language of this area?	Yes / No
3. Are you from this district?	Yes / No
4. How many populations are in your catchment area? ....|_____|	
5. Opening hours of AN clinic: Days/month |_____| Hours/day |_____|	
6. How many of pregnant women in your catchment area come for ANC in one month? (approximate)...|_____|	
7. What are the reason for coming for antenatal care? (asking for her opinion)	
8. What are the reasons for not coming to this ANC/delivery care service? What do you think?	
9. Do you think the catse system in this area influence use of ANC/delivery care services? Please explain.	
10. Is service for normal delivery available - at night? .... |____| -at weekend? .... |____| 11. Is service for care of complicated delivery available -at night? ..|____| -at weekend? ..|____|	
IST on safe motherhood, ANC, delivery care, post-natal care.	
Do you have **supervision** form ? Did doctor or nurse or from DHO office come for supervision in the last 12 months?	
How many times were during the last 12 months?	
Did you (or other person from this PHC/HP) have supervisory visit to the health post/sub-health post/tTBA within the catchment area during the last 12 months?	

CONTENTS OF ANTENATAL AND OBSTETRIC CARE (to ANM/MCHW)			
What will you do, if you see a pregnant women has the following single condition? (score 16/n)			
Condition	nothing special	advice hospital delivery	prompt referral to hospital
1. she is in her first pregnancy			
2. she had operation with previous delivery			
3. she is very short			
4. she is very tall			
5. she has severe headache with blurred vision			
6. she is < 19 years old			
7. she had stillbirth with previous delivery			
8. she has vaginal bleeding			
9. she has lost of consciousness			
10. she has 3 previous pregnancies			
11. she has only daughters			
12. she had severe bleeding in previous delivery			
13. she has limping foot			
14. baby is breech presentation after 36 weeks of pregnancy			
15. she has twin pregnancy			
16. she is 25 years old			

What do you do, if a pregnant woman had a stillbirth in her last pregnancy?
  check VDRL (1)
  advice/refer for hospital delivery (1)
 	
Which BP value should not be exceeded in a pregnant woman ? (1)
  140/90
 	
How do you calculate the EDD ? (1)
  demonstration of correct use of gravidogram or
  date of LMP - 3 months + 7 days or
  today's date + (40 - fundal height in cm) x weeks
 	
When is the time a women should start breast feeding? (1)
  1 hour after delivery

What are the steps you perform in care of normal delivery?
  1. looking at ANC card
  2. using partograph
  3. check completeness of placenta
  4. drying new-born and keeping warm
  5. assessing Apgar score
  6. clear airway if needed
  7. breast feeding within 1 hour
  8. monitoring uterine retraction
  9. monitoring PP blood loss

What do you do, if a baby is not breathing well 1 minute after delivery ? (score 4/n)
  Dry him and keep him warm (1)
  Suction mouth and nostrils (1)
  Stimulate breathing by flickering the baby's sole (1)
  If not improving: ventilate with bag and mask or mouth to mouth, external cardiac massage if heartbeat slow or absent (1)

What would you do if a women in labour can not deliver after 12 hours the onset of labour pain? (score 6/n)
  1. assess mother vital sign (T, pulse, BP, dehydration)
  2. assess lie/presentation/engagement
  3. assess foetal heart
  4. empty bladder
  5. give antibiotics
  6. referral

What do/will you do if a woman has severe bleeding after placenta has been expelled completely? (score 6/n)
  1. assess women's vital sign/condition (1)
  2. establish i.v. line (1)
  3. massage uterus /bimanual compression of uterus (1)
  4. give oxytocics (1)
  5. empty bladder (1)
  6. arrange for emergency referral (1)

Do this center offer/do AN health education session? ....|____| How many sessions were hold in the last 3 or 6 months? .... |____|
TBAs (to ask the personnel who is concern with supervision of TBA)
- concerned person for supervision of tTBAs:
- number of trained TBAs are there in your catchment area:
- number of pregnant women cared by one tTBA during the last 3 months: -number of deliveries done by one tTBA in the last 12 months:
- number of cases refered by TBAs to this center during the last 12 months:
Are they provided with TBA kit box? Is this kit refilled?   By whom? Are they provided the clean home delivery kit (sutkari Samagri)? Is sutkari samagri available in medical shop here or at this facility?

Annexes

Annex 6: Questionnaire for antenatal exit interview

ID no._____

Explain the purpose of study and ask the women for permission verbally.
Assurance of confidentiality will be given verbally.

	Date month year
Date of interview:..|___|___|___|	
Place of interview: (name of HC[1]) _____	
Name of interviewer:_____	

Ask the women for AN card and look for the followings questions. If there is no card, ask the women except questions number _____ .

1. Name:............................... Registration number: ....
2. Age (YEARS) ....|___|
3. Place of residence:............................. urban/rural) ....
4. Religion: _____
5. Ethnicity: _____
6. No. of pregnancies (gestations) .... |___|
7. No of abortions: ....|___|
8. No of stillbirths: ....|___|
9. Uterine height at the first AN visit (or by uterine height): ....|___|
(How long was your pregnancy when you come first?)
10.Number of AN visits (including today visit) ....|___|
(How many time have you come for ANC in this pregnancy for ANC?)
11.Months of pregnancy by now: ....|___|
12.Fe/folic acid prescribed: ....|___|
(1 = Yes, 2 = No, 3 = not recorded/ not known)
13.Tetanus toxoid given with this pregnancy: ....|___|
(1 = Yes, 2 = No, 3 = not recorded/ not known)
Number of TT doses: (1 or 2 doses) ....|___|
(did you get injection at your arm in this pregnancy? How many?)

---

[1] HC = Primary Health Centres/Health Post/Sub-Health Post

14. Risk factors noted: ....|___| (1 = Yes, 2 = not recorded) If yes, reason/s:
15. Delivery at hospital advised: ....|___| (1 = Yes, 2 = not recorded) If Yes, reason for advice: _____

Ask the women the following questions

16. How long did it take you come to the clinic? ....|___| (For ONE Way in Hours)

17. How did you travel to come to this HC? ....|___|
    1. on foot
    2. by bicycle
    3. by bus
    4. by tempo
    5. by rickshaw
    6. by tanga
    7. others (specify)............................

18. How much did you pay for transport? ....Rs. |___| 0.00= no payment
19. Why do you choose this HC (place)?
20. What was the main reason for coming for ANC?
21. How long did you wait before your consultation? (minutes/hours). |___| Is it ....|___| (1 = too long, 2 = it is OK, 3 = no idea, 4 = no answer)

Annexes

For First Time Visit With This Pregnancy, go to number 23 .

Explanation: Now let's talk about the previous AN visit.
22. Did the health worker ask you to buy iron/folate in your previous ANC visit? (vitamin for better health and blood) .... |____| (1 = Yes, 2 = No, 3 = No answer, 4 = don't know)   Have you bought it? ....|____| (1 = Yes, 2 = No, 3 = No answer)   If Yes, Rs. ....   If No, why?...   Did you take all the Fe/folate you bought? (Y/N)   ....|____|

23. Did you get advice from this service about ......
   1. what food to eat ....|____|
   2. danger signs during pregnancy and childbirth ....|____|
   3. how to take the medicine you bought ....|____|
   4. birth spacing/control ....|____|
 (1= yes, 2 = no, 3 = don't remember, 4 = no answer, 5 = not applicable)
 If number (2) is Yes, What danger signs did they tell you?
 ....

24. Did you get a chance to ask question during your consultation? .|____| (1 = yes, 2 = no, 3 = no question to ask)
Now let's talk about your delivery.
25. Did the HW talk with you about the place for your delivery? ...|____| (1 = yes, 2 = no, 3 = don't remember, 4 = no answer)

26. Where do you intend to deliver your baby? ....|____|
     1. at government health facility
     2. at private health facility
     3. at your home
     4. at your relative house in town
     5. maternal waiting home
     6. not known yet
     7. others (specify) _____

27. Why do you intend to deliver in that place? (WAIT FOR SPONTANEOUS ANSWER)...	
28. Did they ask to come back for follow up? ....|____| (1 = yes, 2 = no, 3 = don't remember, 4 = no answer) If yes, reason?	
29. Will you come back? ....|____| (1 = yes, 2 = no, 3 = don't know yet, 4 = no answer) If yes or no, Why?	

30. What do you think about this service? Do you like
  1. attitude of staff ....|____|
  2. examination done ....|____|
  3. explanation of about your pregnancy ....|____|
  4. instruction about medicine ....|____|
  (1 = yes, 2 = no, 3 = don't know, 4 = no answer)	

31. How many times a pregnant women should come for ANC in one pregnancy? {minimum number} ....|____| What benefits do you get from AN check up?	
32. How many TT injection you should get in one pregnancy? ...|____| What is the benefits of that TT injection?	
33. How much do you pay for service fees? (first time visit)   Rs._____
34. How much do you pay for service fees? (more visit)   Rs._____
35. How much do you pay for TT injection?   Rs._____
36. What suggestion do you want to give for improvement of this service? ....

Annexes

Annex 7: Questionnaire for hospital maternity interview

ID no._____

Explain the purpose of study and ensure confidentiality.

Date of interview: ....Date-Month-Year _____
Name of interviewer:_____

The followings are to be filled from in-patient chart or ask the women if data are not available

1. Name:	Registration number:
2. Age: _____ years	
3. Place of residence: (enter name of the village/town) (in Km)	
4. Religion: _____	
5. Ethnicity: _____	
6. No of pregnancies: _____ (enter number)	
7. No of abortions: _____	
8. No of stillbirths: _____ (birth of dead baby)	
9. Time of admission: _____ (enter date/month/year) _____ (enter time in hours/minutes)	
10. Time of attendance by the health personnel⊗date/month/year) _____ (hour/minute) _____	
11. Mode of delivery: ...._____ 12. Normal vaginal delivery 13. CS², emergency 14. CS, planned 15. forceps/vacuum extraction 16. breech delivery 17. twin delivery 7. others _____	
12. Outcome of the baby: ☐ alive ☐ stillbirth weight: _____ gm	

---

² CS = Caesarean Section

Only for C-section/ operative delivery (number _____)

13. Time of decision for C-section/operative delivery (date and time)	
14. Time of C-section /0perative delivery (date and time)	
15. Reason for operation	
16. Condition of the mother: ....□ T > 38 C more than 24 hours	

The followings are to ask all women

17. Did you go for ANC in this pregnancy? Yes/No
Yes --- do not ask _26_ . No --- Go to _26_.
18. Number of ANC visit with this pregnancy?....................|___|
19. Fe tablet prescribed by HW during ANC? Yes/No
No --- **Go to 21.**
20. Days of Fe tablets taken during this pregnancy? ....|___|
21. Number TT dose with this pregnancy? ....|___|
22. Did the health worker advice you to deliver in the hospital? Yes/No
No ------ go to _27_.
23. What was the reason for that advice?
24. When did you get that advice?
25. During ANC ... **If (1), go to number 28**
26. During delivery. ... **If (2), go to number 25**
27. Date and time of that advice? ...._____
(ONLY FOR ADVICE DURING DELIVERY)
26. What was the reasons for not going to the ANC?
27. What reasons made you to come to the hospital?

28. How did you come to the hospital? ....|___|
   1. by rickshaw
   2. by tempo
   3. by bus
   4. others (specify) ....

29. How much did you pay for transport? .... Rs. |_____|

30. How much have you spend after coming to this hospital?

    for operation/delivery: Rs._____

    for medications: Rs._____

    for buying materials: Rs._____

    others (specify)_____ Rs._____

    TOTAL: Rs. _____

31. Were you advice for birth spacing/sterilisation? ....|____|

    (during ANC)

Thank you very much for your co-operation.

Annex 8: Guideline for focus group discussions

1. What women in this village normally would do when she notice that she is pregnant?
    (probe: traditional beliefs and practice, modern antenatal care)

2. Some women go to health services for care of pregnancy, others not. What is your opinion?
    Different kind of care available for care during pregnancy, reasons for use and non-use of these services.

3. Some women give child birth with the help of trained person from health services or trained TBA for childbirth, others not. What is your opinion?
    Different kind of care available for childbirth, reasons for use and non-use, prefer place and assistant for childbirth.
    (probe: alone, mother-in-law, grand mother, TBAs, traditional healers, modern health workers)

4. Some women were asked to go to hospital during pregnancy or for giving birth for different reasons. Some go, but sometimes, they themselves or their relatives refuse to go. Why? What is your opinion?

5. Where do women or their family ask for help in case of problems or complications during pregnancy and childbirth?
    Place, person and reason for choice.
    In case of previous delivery of dead baby.
    In case of labour longer than 12 hours and the baby can not be delivered.
    In case of a lot of bleeding before childbirth.
    In case of a lot of bleeding after delivery.
    In case when women get convulsion.
    In case when women has high fever with bad smelling vaginal discharge.
    In case of Bhiringi.

Annex 9: Guideline for key-informant interviews

1. Some women go to health services for care of pregnancy, others not. What is your opinion?
2. Some women give child birth with the help of trained person from health services or trained TBA for childbirth, others not. What is your opinion?
3. Some women were asked to go to hospital during pregnancy or for giving birth for different reasons. Some go, but sometimes, they themselves or their relatives refuse to go. Why? What is your opinion?

Annexes

Annex 10: Indicators for assessment of antenatal and obstetric care services at a district level

1. General Indicators for Antenatal and Obstetric Care

	Indicators	• Definition	Source
	Availability of services		
1.	- total facilities static facilities - mobile service outlets	• static HCs offering ANC per population) • outreach points which offer ANC (at least monthly) per population	DPHO office
2.	- traditional birth attendants (TBA)	• Trained TBA[1] per population • Trained TBA per expected pregnancy • proportion of villages covered by trained TBA	DPHO office
3.	- trained staff[2] (ANM & staff nurse, MCHW)	• Trained {female}[3] staff entitled for ANC per population in public services • $\dfrac{\#^{4}\ HC\ with\ trained\ \{female\}\ staff}{\#\ total\ HC\ in\ the\ district} \times 100$ • Trained midwife/staff nurse for maternity care per population (public services)	DPHO office
4.	knowledge of staff (FLHS & Hospital)	• proportion of correct answers in a short knowledge test on ANC and delivery care by FLHS staff • proportion of correct answers in a short knowledge test on delivery care by hospital staff	Staff interview
5.	- facility, equipment, drugs, & consumable	• score achieved by FLHS in "essential equipment, drugs and consumable checklist" • score achieved by hospital labour room & theatre in "equipment, essential drugs and consumable checklist"	Facility checklist

---

[1] Trained TBA = lay person providing delivery assistance and got training from formal health service
[2] Trained staff = according to national guideline
[3] female staff = should be change according to culture
[4] # = number of

	Accessibility of services		
6.	- geographical accessibility	• population living within 5 ,6-10, > 10 km from HC -------------------------------- x 100 total population in area assessed	VDC office of sample
7.	- seasonal accessibility	population cut off from access to NG (by flooding etc.) for >=1 month/year -------------------------------- X 100 total population in the district	DPHO office
	Process quality		
8.	- co-operation with TBA	• # referrals (both ante and intra-partum) received from TBA in last 3 months -------------------------------------- x 4 # expected pregnancy in HC catchment area • # HC supplying/refilling the TBA' delivery kits -------------------------------------- # HC assessed • # refresher training with TBA in last year -------------------------------- x 100% # TBA in HC catchment area (265)	HW interview
9.	- supervision received (by HW)	• # supervisory contact concerning ANC [and delivery care] received from higher level in last year ---------------------------------- x 100% # HC assessed	HW interview
	supervision given to TBA	• # supervisory contact concerning ANC [and delivery care] given to TBA by HW in last year -------------------------------- x 100% # HC assessed	HW interview

	Output		
10.	- institutional delivery rate	# delivery in institution / # expected deliveries/district/year × 100	birth register
11.	- community-based C-section rate	(# C-sections performed at hospital & private + # women referred for C-section elsewhere) / # expected deliveries in the district × 100	operation register

2. Indicators for preventive and promotive ANC activities for all pregnant women

	Availability of ANC		
12.	- consultations hours	average hours & days per month during which ANC is offered at each HC	observation
13.	- examinations	# HC able to measure BP on day of observation / # HCs assessed × 100	observation
	Accessibility of ANC		
14.	- financial accessibility	direct costs[4] of 3 ANC visits for the client legal minimum daily wage • cost for consultation • cost for medicine	exit interview
15.	- cultural/ communicative	# ANC providers speaking the local language / total # ANC providers interviewed × 100	HW interview & observation
	Process quality of ANC		
16.	- waiting time	avge waiting time for ANC attendee from arrival at HC until her individual consultation begins # ANC attendees complaining of waiting too long / # ANC attendees interviewed × 100	exit interview
17.	- individual consultation time	avge duration of individual consultations in min	observation

18.	- individual counselling time	• avge time spent on individual counselling in min	observation
19.	- contents of counselling	• avge score n/18 for contents of counselling: • education about cleanliness (2), about nutrition (2), enquiry about woman's social situation (2) place of delivery (2) information on family planning methods (2) when to seek medical care in pregnancy (p.v.-bleeding, severe headache/visual disturbances, convulsions, pallor, fever, labour > 12h [1 p. each sign]) (6) • assurance of women (2)	observation
Output of ANC			
20.	- "crude" coverage of ANC (district)	• # first ANC visits in last year (HP/SHP/Hospital/private) ----------------------------------- x 100 expected # deliveries in HC catchment pop. / year	ANC register, (district)
21.	- crude coverage (sampled)	• as above stratified for population <=5km and >5km [or 1 hour walking time] from HC (only FLHS)	ANC register, FLHS
22.	- "valid" coverage	• proportion of women with >= 3 visits X "crude" coverage	-ditto-
23.	- intensity of use	• total # ANC consultation --------------- in last year (only FLHS) # first ANC visits	-ditto-
24.	- timeliness of ANC	• # 1st visits within 20 [36] weeks after LMP ---------------------------------- x 100 # first ANC visits	-ditto-
25.	- productivity	• # ANC consultations in last year (1st+repeat) -------------------------------------- # ANC clinic hrs x # staff on duty at each clinic day	-ditto- & HW interview

26.	- anaemia prophylaxis prescription rate	• # ANC attendees/maternity cases having received [a prescription of] Fe/Folate ---------------------------------- x 100 # ANC attendees/maternity cases interviewed	ANC exit & maternity interviews
27.	- compliance with anaemia prophylaxis	• # women reporting to have actually taken all the tablets of Fe received ---------------------------------- x 100 # women >2 visit & received iron tablet	ANC exit
28.	- intensity of anaemia prophylaxis	• # women who took >=30 days Fe tablets x 100 • # women who received Fe tablet	maternity interview
29.	- effective coverage	• # women taking >=30 days Fe tablets x 100 • # expected deliveries	ANC exit & maternity interviews
30.	- coverage[5] with TT immunization (proxy)[6]	• # women who got >= 2 doses of TT in last year ---------------------------------- x 100 # target women for TT	monthly reports
31.	- coverage[7] with TT immunization (proxy)[8]	• # women who received >= 2 dose of TT during this pregnancy ---------------------------------- x 100 # ANC women interviewed	ANC exit
32.	- valid coverage with TT immunization	• # women who had been vaccinated with 2 doses TT by the time of delivery[9] ---------------------------------- x 100 # maternity interview	maternity
33.	- health education coverage	• % of HC holding health education class for ANC attendees	HW interview
		• # women reporting to have received information on '*' during ANC ---------------------------------- x 100 # women interviewed	Exit interview

---

[5] as a proportion of all ANC attenders
[6] indicator has to be modified, if there is a sizable proportion of women immunized prior to present pregnancy
[7] as a proportion of all ANC attenders
[8] indicator has to be modified, if there is a sizable proportion of women immunized prior to present pregnancy
[9] according to WHO/GPV guidelines

		• ---- on danger signs -------	-ditto-
		• ---- on nutrition----	-ditto-
		• ----- on family planning---	-ditto-
		• -- place of delivery---	
34.	- effectiveness of health education	•# women who can reproduce information on *at least one danger sign* told -- x 100 # all women interviewed	ANC exit
		•# women who knows the benefit of TT injection x 100 / # women interviewed	-ditto-
35.	- coverage with family planning advice	•# women reporting to have received family planning advice during ANC -- x 100 # women interviewed	maternity interview

3. Indicators for screening in ANC

Process quality			
36.	- completeness of history taking at first visit	• proportion of items asked (1 score each): age, marital status, village, parity, number of living children, stillbirths, abortions, any complications in previous deliveries, any previous major illnesses, STDs symptoms, current complaints	observation
37.	- completeness of physical examination	• proportion of examinations correctly performed, expressed as score : maternal height (1), BP (1), clinical pallor (1), fundal height (1), foetal heart (1), presentation of foetus (GA > 32 weeks) (1)	observation
38.	population-based detection rate	• # pregnancies identified as "at risk" --------------------------------- x 100 expected frequency of at risk pregnancies in the population x n n = number of women screened	ANC register
		• --- previous SB-----	
		• --- short stature -----	
		• ----hypertension-----	
		• ----twin ----	
		• ----breech -----	
		• ----anaemia ----	

Annexes

39.	- correct interpretation of signs detected	• # pregnancies identified as "at risk" due to *short maternal stature* ---------------------------------- x 100 # ANC attendees documented to be smaller than cut off point acc. to NG	ANC register
		• # pregnancies identified as "at risk" due to *hypertension* ---------------------------- x 100 # ANC attendees documented to have BP > 140/90	
		• ----young age----	
		• ----primi----	
40.	- correct interpretation of anamnestic risk factors	• # pregnancies identified as "at risk" due to *multiparity* -------------------------------- x 100 # ANC attenders qualifying as multips acc. To NG (G4 +)	ANC register at HC
		• # pregnancies identified as "at risk" due to *previous stillbirth / PPH / C-section* ------------------------- x 100 # ANC attenders documented to have had previous stillbirth /PPH / C-section	
Output of screening			
41.	- proportion of referral advice	• # pregnant women who are advised to go to hospital for consultation and/or for delivery due to a risk factor detected during ANC -------------------------------- x 100 # total attendees	ANC register
42.	- proportion of referral in hospital	• # women delivered at the hospital due to referral advice by HW --------------------------- x 100 # maternity interviewed	maternity interview
43.	- coverage of antenatally referral advice for high risk pregnancy	• # pregnant women who are advised to go to hospital for consultation and/or for delivery due to a risk factor detected during ANC --------------------------- x 100 # expected pregnancies of accumulation of high risk pregnancies	ANC register, HC staff

4. Indicators for delivery care at health centre level

	Availability		
44.	- Availability of delivery care	• hours x days per week during which a trained midwife is on call at HC	HC staff
	Process quality		
45.	- description of routine delivery care & neonatal care FLHS: Hospital:	• score n/10 for mentioning: • looking at ANC card, using partograph, assessing APGAR, drying new born, keeping new born warm, clear airways if necessary, breast feeding within 1 hr after birth, check completeness of placenta, monitoring postpartal contraction of uterus, monitoring postpartal blood loss	HC staff interview[10]
46.	monitoring of labour	• # deliveries with correct partograph -------------------------- x 100 # deliveries at HC	HC delivery records
47.	- completeness of documentation	• avge # categories filled in birth register -------------------------- x 100 # categories provided in birth register	HC birth register
	Output		
48.	- proportion of assisted deliveries	• # of deliveries at HC[11] [+# home deliveries conducted by trained midwives] -------------------------- x 100 expected # deliveries in HC catchment population	HW interview
	- same stratified by distance from HC	• # of deliveries at HC in women living <=5 / 5-10 / > 10 km from the HC -------------------------- x 100 expected # deliveries in respective population	HC birth register, district map
49.	- emergency referral ratio	• # intrapartum[12] referrals actually taking place to higher level -------------------------- x 100 # deliveries at HC	HC birth registers

---

[10] relying on what the staff reports as their normal practice as it is logistically very difficult to directly observe a sufficient number of deliveries at HC level
[11] excluding women who arrive at HC after the baby or the first twin has already been born
[12] intrapartum referral = woman who intended to deliver at home or in a HC and in whom the decision for referral was made during delivery

Annexes

	Outcome		
50.	- ratio of stillbirths at HC	• # SB >= 2000g / # deliveries at HC x 100	HC birth register
51.	- ratio of neonatal deaths	• # early neonatal deaths[13] / # deliveries at HC x 100	HC birth register
52.	- maternal mortality ratio	• # maternal deaths[11] / # deliveries at HC x 100	HC birth register

5. Indicators for referral advice

	Accessibility of referral level obstetric care		
53.	- geographical	• distance to hospital from furthest villages of the district in km [in travel time]	district map / DMO's
		• population within * km of hospital / total district population x 100	district map / DMO's office
		• # HC where transport to hospital is available / total # HC x 100	HC staff / DMO's office
		• travel time by car (range / mean) between HC and hospital	HC staff / DPHO
54.	- financial	• cost of transport to hospital for the client (range / mean for all HC assessed) in local currency [in DM]	maternity inpatient interviews
		• mean cost of transport to hospital for client / daily wage of unskilled labourer	maternity inpatient interviews
		• mean cost of vaginal delivery / daily wage of unskilled labourer	-ditto------
		• cost of caesarean section incl. Post-op treatment for the client / daily wage of unskilled labourer	-- ditto-----

---

[13] deaths occuring while still admitted at HC (state normal period of stay)

#			
55.	- access to hospital in emergencies	• # stillbirths in hospital in women living <=30km / >30km from hospital ------------------------------------- x 100 # hospital deliveries in women living <=30km / >30km from hospital	hospital birth register / district population
		# extra-uterine pregnancy seen at the hospital/ year ------------------------------------- x 100 expected ratio in the population x district population	enumerator: hospital theatre book denominator
56.	- delay	• average time interval between referral recommendation and actual arrival at hospital (intrapartum referrals)	HC staff interviews / maternity inpatient interviews
Output with respect to referral			
57.	- population-based referral advice rate	• referral advice rate from ANC x ANC coverage	ANC register
58.	- population based actual referral rate	• institutional delivery rate x % women referred	
	- same stratified by distance of home place from hospital	• # all referred women living {<= 10km /11-30km / 31 km +} from the hospital ------------------------------- x 100 # expected deliveries in population {<=10km /11-30km / 31 km +} from the hospital	maternity interviews / district population
59.	- proportion of referred women in hospital deliveries	• # all referred women delivering at hospital ------------------------------- x 100 # deliveries at the hospital	maternity interview
	- proportion of *antepartum* referrals[14]	• # women referred antepartum ------------------------------- x 100 # deliveries at the hospital	-ditto-

---

[14] antepartum referral = woman who comes to hospital for consultation and/or delivery because she has been told so during ANC. She may be in labour upon admission, provided she did not intend to deliver on a lower level.

Annexes

	- proportion of *emergency* referrals[15]	• # women referred intrapartum -------------------------- x 100 # deliveries at the hospital	-ditto-
60.	- antepartum referral compliance	• antenatally referral cases in hospital deliveries x 100 --- estimated total referral advice from the district	maternity interview
61.	- intrapartum referral compliance	• # women actually arriving at hospital for delivery after intrapartum referral from HC --- x 100 # intrapartum referrals recommended in HC	ANC register/ maternity register
62.	- proportion of risk pregnancies among hospital deliveries	• # women delivered in hospital with risk factor ---------------------------------- x 100 # deliveries in hospital	hospital births register
		• ---primi-	
		• ---age <19 yr-	
		• ---multip (G4 +)-	
		• ---previous SB-	
		• ---breech-	
		• ---twin-	
63.	- community-based caesarean section rate	• # C-sections performed at hospital + # women referred for C-section elsewhere -------------------------------------- x 100 # expected deliveries in the district	theatre register/ district population
64.	profile of indications for C-section	• # C-sections due to indication X ---------------------------------- x 100 # total C-sections	theatre / maternity register
		• ---CPD & obstructed labour-	
		• ---abnormal lie & presentation-	
		• ---APH-	
		• ---previous CS-	
		• ---PET & eclampsia-	
		• ---foetal distress & others-	

---

[15] intrapartum referral = woman who intended to deliver at home or in a HC and in whom the decision for referral was made during delivery

| 65. | - proportion of emergency C-sections[16] | • # emergency C-sections $\frac{\text{\# emergency C-sections}}{\text{\# total C-sections}} \times 100$ | theatre/birth register |

6. Indicators for referral level obstetric care

Availability of referral level obstetric care			
66.	- facility	• catchment population of referral centres	DMO's office
67.	- trained staff	• # trained midwives in hospital maternity	DMO/ observation at hospital
		• # surgeons or other staff performing caesarean sections	DMO/ observation at hospital
68.	- availibility of essential elements of obstetric care as defined by WHO	• score n/16[17] on the day of assessment: surgical obstetrics, anaesthesia, medical treatment, blood transfusion, manual procedure and continuous monitoring of labour by qualified staff, management of women at high risk, family planning, neonatal care	observation at hospital (checklist)
69.	- continuity of referral level obstetric care	• days per week and hours per day during which theatre is able to perform C-section	hospital staff / observation
		• # women referred for C-section elsewhere $\frac{\text{\# women referred for C-section elsewhere}}{\text{\# total decisions for C-section}} \times 100$	birth register / maternity patient register
70.	- continuity of blood supply	• # days on which blood was available in last year $\frac{\text{\# days on which blood was available in last year}}{365 \text{ days}} \times 100$	hospital staff interviews

---

[16] emergency C-section = caesarean section for which the decision was made during delivery (as opposed to elective C-section)

[17] 2 points = item is fully and rapidly available, 1 = partially available or available with delay, 0 = not available

Annexes

	Process quality		
71.	- completeness of examination on admission (proxy)	• score n/16:[21] • ask for current complaints (2), obstetric history incl. present pregnancy (2), blood pressure/ maternal pulse (2), pallor (2), duration and frequency of contractions (2), presentation of foetus (2), foetal heart rate (2), cervical dilatation (2),	staff interview
72.	- care of normal delivery (proxy)	• similar to FLHS interview	staff interview
73.	- post delivery care for the mother (proxy)	• score n/10 :[18] monitoring uterine contraction (2), monitoring postpartal blood loss (2), daily BP and temperature (2), breast feeding support (2), family planning advice (2)	hospital staff interviews
74.	- routine new born care (proxy)	• score n/10 :[21] check APGAR (2), keep baby dry and warm (2), breast feeding within 1 hr of delivery (2), apply silver nitrate (or antibiotic) eye drops (2), rooming in (2)	hospital staff interviews / observation
75.	- monitoring of labour	• # deliveries in which partograph has been employed correctly ------------------------------x 100 # delivery records checked	check 20 delivery records
76.	- swiftness of emergency interventions	• preparation time for caesarean section [day / night]	theatre staff interviews
		• time lapse between decision for and actual time of CS	maternity interview
		• time lapse between admission and attendance by staff	-ditto-

---

[18] scoring: 2 points = carried out correctly, 1 = carried out with shortcomings, 0 = not done

	Output		
77.	- ratio of caesarean sections in hospital	• # C-sections (elective / emergency) ------------------------------- x 100 # deliveries in hospital	hospital birth register
78.	- ratio of vacuum extractions / forceps / symphysiotomies in hospital	• # forceps ------------------- x 100 # deliveries in hospital	hospital birth register
	Outcome		
79.	- ratio of stillbirths in hospital	• # SB ------------------------ x 100 # deliveries in hospital	hospital register
		• ----- >= 2500 gm -------	hospital register
80.	- ratio of stillbirths after C-section	• # C-sections resulting in stillbirth ------------------------------- x 100 # C-sections	hospital register
81.	- neonatal mortality of babies <2500g in hospital	• # neonatal deaths in babies <2500g -------------------------------- x 100 # total babies <2500g born in hospital	hospital register
82.	- maternal mortality in hospital	• # maternal deaths in hospital --------------------------- x 100000 # total hospital deliveries	hospital register
83.	- maternal mortality after caesarean section	• # maternal deaths after C-section --------------------------- x 100000 # C-sections	hospital register

MEDIZIN IN ENTWICKLUNGSLÄNDERN

Schriftenreihe zur Medizin und zu Gesundheitsproblemen in Ländern der Dritten Welt

Band 1 Wolfgang Bichmann: Die Problematik der Gesundheitsplanung in Entwicklungsländern. Ein Beitrag zur Geschichte, der Situation und den Perspektiven der Planung des nationalen Gesundheitswesens in den > Least Developed Countries < Afrikas. 1979.

Band 2 Jens Herrmann: Ambition and Reality - Planning for Health and Basic Health Services in the Yemen Arab Republic. 1979.

Band 3 J.M. Pönninghaus: The Cost Benefit of Measles Immunisation. A Study from Southern Zambia. 1979.

Band 4 Hilde Wander (Hrsg.): Bedingungen und Möglichkeiten der Integrierung bevölkerungspolitischer Programme in die nationale und die internationale Entwicklungspolitik. 1980.

Band 5 M. Heidegger/H.J. Diesfeld/A. Selheim: Demographische und soziale Wirkungen von Familienplanung. 1980.

Band 6 H.J. Diesfeld (Hrsg.): Importierte Krankheiten und ärztliche Untersuchungen vor und nach Tropenaufenthalt. Kongreßbericht über die X. Tagung der Deutschen Tropenmedizinischen Gesellschaft vom 22.-24. März 1979 in Heidelberg. 1980.

Band 7 Alexander Boroffka: Benedict Nta Tanka's Commentary and Dramatized Ideas on "Disease and Witchcraft in our Society". A Schreber Case from Cameroon Annotated Autobiographical Notes by an African on his Mental Illness. 1980.

Band 8 Hartmut Brandt: Work Capacity Restraints in Tropical Agricultural Development. 1980.

Band 9 nicht erschienen

Band 10 Tilman Nitzschke / Donata von Lüttwitz: Annehmbarkeit präventiver und promotiver Maßnahmen eines Health Centre für die Bevölkerung. Dargestellt am Beispiel der ländlichen Gesundheitsversorgung der Vereinigten Republik Kamerun. 1981.

Band 11 H.J. Diesfeld (Ed.): Health Research in Developing Countries. Proceedings of the Joint Meeting of the Belgische Vereniging voor Tropische Geneeskunde, Societé Belge de Medecine Tropicale, the Nederlandse Vereniging voor Tropische Geneeskunde and the Deutsche Tropenmedizinische Gesellschaft. 1982.

Band 12 Axel Kroeger/Francoise Barbira-Freedman: Cultural Change and Health: The Case of Southamerican Rainforest Indians. With special reference to the Shuar/Achuar of Ecuador. 1982.

Band 13 Dorothea Sich: Mutterschaft und Geburt im Kulturwandel. Ein Beitrag zur transkulturellen Gesundheitsforschung aus Korea. 1982.

Band 14 Uwe K. Brinkmann: Onchozerkose in Westafrika. 1982.

Band 15 Peter Oberender/Hans Jochen Diesfeld/Wolfgang Gitter (Hrsg.): Health and Development in Africa. International, Interdisciplinary Symposium, 2-4 June 1982, University of Bayreuth. 1983.

Band 16 Josef Boch (Hrsg.): Tropenmedizin, Parasitologie, Trypanosomiasis, Malaria, Bilharziose, Onchozerkose, Importierte Virusinfektionen, Lepra, Intermediate Technology, Zecken und durch sie übertragene Krankheiten, Immundiagnostik. 1984.

Band 17 Abdin Hamid Shaddad: Anforderungen an Gesundheitseinrichtungen der Basisversorgung im Sudan. Ein Beitrag zur Gesundheitsversorgung und zu baulichen Maßnahmen für die Gesundheitseinrichtungen unter besonderer Berücksichtigung der vorhandenen Ressourcen, der sozialen Verhältnisse und der klimatischen Bedingungen. 1984.

Band 18 Gerhard Heller: Krankheitskonzepte und Krankheitssymptome. Eine empirische Untersuchung bei den Tamang von Cautara/Nepal zur Frage der kulturspezifischen Prägung von Krankheitserleben. 1985.

Band 19 Hans-Jochen Diesfeld / Sigrid Wolter (Hrsg.): Medizin in Entwicklungsländern. Handbuch zur praxisorientierten Vorbereitung für medizinische Entwicklungshelfer. 5. neubearbeitete Auflage. 1989.

Band 20 Verena Kücholl: Soziokulturelle Wege des Heilens. Eine ethnomedizinische Analyse und Interpretation des Samkhya und der Heiltradition der Navajo. 1985.

Band 21 Frank-Peter Schelp (Ed.): Health Problems in Asia and in the Federal Republic of Germany. How to solve them? Proceedings of a seminar on "Techniques and Problems of Intervention Trials in Developing and Developed Countries". 1985.

Band 22 Rolf Heinmüller, Winfried Kern: Primäre Gesundheitsversorgung im südwestlichen Sudan. Eine Feldforschung bei den südsudanesischen Azande zur Evaluierung der Einflüsse des 'Primary Health Care'-Programms auf gesundheitliche Lage und allgemeine Lebensbedingungen. Detailed English Summary. 1987.

Band 23 Andreas Hahold/Axel Kroeger: Krankheitsbewältigung im Andenhochland Perus. Ergebnisse einer Bevölkerungsbefragung. 1986.

Band 24 Georg Kamm / Peter Witton / Hatibu Lweno: Anaesthesia Notebook for Medical Auxilaries. With special Reference to Anaesthesia Practice in Developing Countries. 1989.

Band 25 Alice S. Kuhn: Heiler und ihre Patienten auf dem Dach der Welt. Ladakh aus ethnomedizinischer Sicht. 1988.

Band 26 Wolfgang Bichmann: Community Involvement in Nepal's Health System. A case study of district health services management and the Community Health Leader scheme in Kaski district. 1989.

Band 27 M. Luisa Vázquez / Renate Lipowsky / Axel Kroeger: Malaria und kutane Leishmaniase in Kolumbien. Vorkommen, Volkskonzepte und traditionelle Behandlungsformen. 1989.

Band 28 Heinrich Berg / Axel Kroeger / Carmen Perez-Samaniego / Fernando Malo: Kranke Menschen – krankes Gesundheitswesen? Eine epidemiologische Untersuchung in Nord-Mexiko. 1989.

Band 29 Emmie Ho-Tsui / Margit Urhahn: Medizin und Gesundheitsforschung in Entwicklungsländern. Bibliographie des Instituts für Tropenhygiene 1984-1988. 1991.

Band 30 Thomas Lux: Gespräche mit afrikanischen Krankenpflegern und Heilern. Bilder von Krankheit im Mikrokosmos von Malanville(Benin), 1991.

Band 31 Christopher Knauth: Arzneimittelgebrauch armer Bevölkerungsschichten in städtischen Elendsvierteln Perus. Möglichkeiten und Grenzen der Gesundheitserziehung zum rationalen Arzneimittelgebrauch. 1991.

Band 32 Erhard Hinz: Geomedizinische und biogeographische Aspekte der Krankheitsverbreitung und Gesundheitsversorgung in Industrie- und Entwicklungsländern. 1991.

Band 33 Klaus Hoffmann: Psychiatrie in Afrika. Eine Einführung für Entwicklungshelfer. 1992.

Band 34 Dorothea Sich / Hans Jochen Diesfeld / Angelika Deigner / Monika Habermann (Hrsg.): Medizin und Kultur. Eine Propädeutik für Studierende der Medizin und der Ethnologie mit 4 Seminaren in Kulturvergleichender Medizinischer Anthropologie (KMA). 1993. 2., unveränd. Aufl. 1995.

Band 35 Annette Wiemann-Michaels: Die verhexte Speise. Eine ethnopsychosomatische Studie über das Depressive Syndrom in Nepal. 1994.

Band 36 Christine Loytved: Hebammen in Ozeanien zwischen traditioneller und westlicher Medizin. Weiterbildung traditioneller Hebammen in Westsamoa und Tonga. 1994.

Band 37 Andrea Materlik: Medizinisch-anthropologische Aspekte von Lepra im Amazonas und ihre Bedeutung für die Gesundheitserziehung. 1994.

Band 38 Oliver Razum: Improving Service Quality through Action Research, as applied in the Expanded Programme on Immunization (EPI). 1994.

Band 39 Ulrich Schramm: Einflußfaktoren auf die Akzeptanz von baulichen Anlagen der ländlichen Gesundheitseinheiten in Ägypten. Fallstudie am Beispiel der staatlichen Einheit in Zebeda unter Verwendung der Post-Occupancy Evaluation. 1995.

Band 40 Rainer Sauerborn / Adrien Nougtara / Hans Jochen Diesfeld (Eds.): Recherche sur les systèmes de santé: Le cas de la zone médicale de Solenzo, Burkina Faso. Auteurs: Rainer Sauerborn, Adrien Nougtara, Hans Jochen Diesfeld, Gaston Sorgho, Joseph Bidiga, Lougousse Tiébélessé, Eric Latimer, Roberto Sallier de La Tour, Uwe Brinkmann, Don Shepard. 1995.

Band 41 Rainer Sauerborn / Adrien Nougtara / Hans Jochen Diesfeld (Eds.): Les Côuts Economiques de la Maladie pour les Ménages au Milieu Rural du Burkina Faso. Avec des contributions de Rainer Sauerborn, Adrien Nougtara, Maurice Hien, Issouf Ibrango, Matthias Borchert, Justus Benzler, Eberhard Koob, Hans Jochen Diesfeld. 1996.

Band 42 Erhard Hinz: Helminthiasen des Menschen in Thailand. 1996.

Band 43 Matthias Perleth: Historical Aspects of American Trypanosomiasis (Chagas' Disease). 1997.

Band 44 Christiane Fischer: Über die Effektivität der Dorfgesundheitsarbeiterinnen innerhalb der Nichtregierungsorganisation ACCORD in Tamil Nadu/Südindien. Aktionsforschung im Rahmen der Gesundheitssystemforschung. 1998.

Band 45 Maureen Dar lang: Assessment of antenatal and obstetric care services in a rural district of Nepal. 1999.

Werner Kaltefleiter / Ulrike Schumacher (Eds.)

The Rise of a Multipolar World

Papers presented at the Summer Course 1997 on International Security

Frankfurt/M., Berlin, Bern, New York, Paris, Wien, 1998. 214 pp., 1 fig., 9 tab.
Conflicts, Options, Strategies in a Threatened World.
Edited by Werner Kaltefleiter and Ulrike Schumacher. Vol. 2
ISBN 3-631-33286-6 · pb. DM 65.–*
US-ISBN 0-8204-3592-9

The international system which was characterized by its bipolar structure until the end of the systemic conflict undergoes a process of change. New regional power centres seem to emerge in various parts of the world. Those centres have begun to position themselves in different roles in their regions. China seems to be on its way towards a position as hegemon in the Asia-Pacific region. India is trying to determine its foreign policy under new auspices after the end of the concept of non-aligned states. Brazil seems to be using its geostrategic position to dominate the South American continent. Those are some examples of the change in the international system from bipolarity to multipolarity. In order to restructure the international community, several approaches can be discussed. Will the United States of America be the world's only superpower? Or, will the United Nations be able to provide collective security? The lectures presented at the Summer Course on International Security 1997 attempt to at least partially answer these questions.

Contents: After the end of the systemic conflict regional powers have gained a new role in the international system: among these are India, China, Brazil, and Germany · Methods of conflict resolution by international institutions and democratic control are discussed

Frankfurt/M · Berlin · Bern · New York · Paris · Wien
Distribution: Verlag Peter Lang AG
Jupiterstr. 15, CH-3000 Bern 15
Fax (004131) 9402131
*incl. value added tax
Prices are subject to change without notice.